JIMD Reports
Volume 40

Eva Morava
Editor-in-Chief

Matthias Baumgartner · Marc Patterson ·
Shamima Rahman · Johannes Zschocke
Editors

Verena Peters
Managing Editor

JIMD Reports
Volume 40

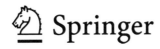 Springer

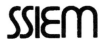

Editor-in-Chief
Eva Morava
Tulane University Medical School
New Orleans
Louisiana
USA

Editor
Marc Patterson
Division of Child and Adolescent Neurology
Mayo Clinic
Rochester
Minnesota
USA

Editor
Johannes Zschocke
Division of Human Genetics
Medical University Innsbruck
Innsbruck
Austria

Editor
Matthias Baumgartner
Division of Metabolism & Children's Research
Centre
University Children's Hospital Zürich
Zürich
Switzerland

Editor
Shamima Rahman
Clinical and Molecular Genetics Unit
UCL Institute of Child Health
London
UK

Managing Editor
Verena Peters
Center for Child and Adolescent Medicine
Heidelberg University Hospital
Heidelberg
Germany

ISSN 2192-8304   ISSN 2192-8312   (electronic)
JIMD Reports
ISBN 978-3-662-57879-7   ISBN 978-3-662-57880-3   (eBook)
https://doi.org/10.1007/978-3-662-57880-3

Contents

JIMD Reports
DOI 10.1007/8904_2017_54

Natural History of Aromatic L-Amino Acid Decarboxylase Deficiency in Taiwan

Wuh-Liang Hwu · Yin-Hsiu Chien · Ni-Chung Lee · Mei-Hsin Li

Received: 20 May 2017 / Revised: 30 July 2017 / Accepted: 10 August 2017 / Published online: 31 August 2017
© Society for the Study of Inborn Errors of Metabolism (SSIEM) 2017

Abstract *Objectives*: Aromatic L-amino acid decarboxylase (AADC) deficiency is a rare inherited disorder of monoamine neurotransmitter synthesis; this deficiency leads to psychomotor delay, hypotonia, oculogyric crises, dystonia, and extraneurological symptoms. This study aimed to provide further insight into the clinical course of AADC deficiency in Taiwan.

Patients and Methods: We present a retrospective, descriptive, single-center study of 37 children with a confirmed diagnosis of AADC deficiency. Their medical histories were reviewed for motor milestones, motor development, *DDC* mutation, and body weight. The termination point for each patient in this study was defined as no further follow-up, death, or enrollment in a gene therapy trial.

Results: The median age of the study patients at the end of the study was 4.39 years (1.28–11.30). Of the 37 patients, 36 did not develop full head control, sitting ability, standing ability, or speech at any time point from birth to the termination points. Motor scales were administered to 22 patients. Their Alberta Infant Motor Scale scores were below the fifth percentile, and their Peabody Developmental Motor Scales, Second Edition, scores were below the first percentile. Their body weights were normal in the first few months of life, but severe growth retardation occurred at later ages. The mutation c.714+4A>T (IVS6+4A>T) accounted for 76% of all their *DDC* mutations.

Conclusion: In this chapter, we report the clinical course of AADC deficiency in Taiwan. Our data will help guide the development of treatment strategies for the disease.

Introduction

Aromatic L-amino acid decarboxylase (AADC, EC 4.1.1.28) deficiency (MIM #608643) is a rare inherited disorder of neurotransmitter synthesis. AADC is responsible for the synthesis of dopamine and serotonin; furthermore, dopamine is the precursor of epinephrine and norepinephrine. AADC deficiency was first identified in 1990 by Hyland and Clayton through screening of cerebrospinal fluid (CSF) samples from children with unidentified neurologic disorders for identifying abnormalities in neurotransmitter metabolites (Hyland and Clayton 1990; Hyland et al. 1992). Currently, approximately 130 patients with AADC deficiency have been reported worldwide according to a recent summary from the International Working Group on Neurotransmitter Related Disorders (Wassenberg et al. 2017). The key symptoms include extreme hypotonia, hypokinesia, oculogyric crises (OGCs), and signs of autonomic dysfunction since early life. However, a few patients with mild or atypical manifestations have also been reported (Graziano et al. 2015; Kojima et al. 2016; Opladen et al. 2016; Spitz et al. 2017).

The prevalence of AADC deficiency is higher in the Chinese population because of the presence of the founder mutation c.714+4A>T (IVS6+4A>T) (Tay et al. 2007; Lee et al. 2009). We previously described the developmental milestones in 20 living patients carrying this prevalent mutation; all patients had typical symptoms of AADC deficiency, and all of them failed to achieve any develop-

Communicated by: Saskia Brigitte Wortmann, M.D., Ph.D.

W.-L. Hwu (✉) · Y.-H. Chien · N.-C. Lee · M.-H. Li
Department of Pediatrics and Medical Genetics, National Taiwan University Hospital and National Taiwan University College of Medicine, Taipei, Taiwan
e-mail: hwuwlntu@ntu.edu.tw

mental milestone despite receiving therapeutic combinations (Hwu et al. 2012). In this chapter, we provide the updated natural history data of 37 patients with AADC deficiency. Moreover, we provide additional information on genotypes, growth, motor developmental milestones, and motor scales to help guide the treatment of the disease in the future.

Methods

In this retrospective, descriptive, single-center study, we explored the natural history of patients who received a diagnosis of AADC deficiency at National Taiwan University Hospital (NTUH), particularly their growth and motor development. Their medical records were reviewed. All patients were followed up by the authors. The diagnoses of AADC deficiency were made based on the presence of a combination of clinical manifestations plus a characteristic CSF neurotransmitter or the presence of two pathogenic DDC mutations. The termination point for each patient in this study was defined as no further follow-up, death, or enrollment in a gene therapy trial. Some patients died at home, and the exact dates of death were not recorded in the medical records. Therefore, the age at death was not known and was excluded from analysis in this study. This study was approved by the Institutional Review Board of NTUH (201303100RIND).

The body weights of patients were retrieved from the medical records for every visit. Moreover, the ages at which the developmental milestones, namely head control, sitting ability, and standing ability, were achieved were obtained from medical histories. The scores in standard motor developmental scales, if performed, were also extracted. The scales used for evaluation included the Alberta Infant Motor Scale (AIMS) and Peabody Developmental Motor Scales, Second Edition (PDMS-2). The AIMS is an observational measure of infant motor performance and can be administered from birth to the age at which independent walking occurs (Darrah et al. 2014). It assesses the sequential development of motor milestones. The PDMS-2 is a skill-based measure of gross and fine motor development for infants and children, and it is administered from 6 months to 6 years of age; it consists of four gross motor and two fine motor subtests. Body weight at each visit was plotted according to age, with respect to the body weight distribution of normal female children (Chen and Chang 2010). The AIMS score was also plotted according to age, in comparison with the fifth percentile of normal children (Darrah et al. 2014).

Results

Demographic Data

Through medical history review, we identified 37 patients who received a diagnosis of AADC deficiency from 2004 to 2016 (Table 1). All patients presented with hypotonia, hypokinesia, and dystonia, and all but patient No. 37 had OGCs. Two DDC mutations were identified in 36 patients, and one mutation was identified in patient No. 37. All patients showed decreased CSF homovanillic acid (HVA) and 5-hydroxyindoleacetic acid (5-HIAA) levels or elevated 3-O-methyldopa (3-OMD) levels in dried blood spots. The termination point for 15 patients was their latest visit, and the termination point for the remaining 22 patients was the last visit before entering a gene therapy trial. The median age of patients at the end of this study was 4.39 years (range: 1.28–11.30). The median age of patients at their first visit to NTUH was 1.10 years (range: 0–7.31), and the median follow-up period was 2.64 years (range: 0–9.34). Three patients (patient No. 10, 21, and 25) were diagnosed through newborn screening; therefore, they visited NTUH shortly after birth. Other patients were referred to NUTH for undiagnosed neurological conditions or for treatment or a second opinion after the diagnosis of AADC deficiency. All patients were ethnically Chinese, except that the ethnicity of patient No. 8 was found to be one-half Caucasian, one-quarter Chinese, and one-quarter Thai.

Mutations

The sequence status of the DDC gene was available for all 37 patients. For all patients, DDC mutations were detected using Sanger sequencing. The most common mutation IVS6+4A>T represented 76% of all DDC mutations (56 of 74 mutated chromosomes), followed by c.1297dupA (p. I433Nfs*60) (5 of 74 mutated chromosomes or 6.8%) and c.1234C>T (p.R412W) (3 of 74 mutated chromosomes or 4.0%). Other mutations included one small deletion and eight rare mutations. Only one mutation was found in patient No. 37 after Sanger sequencing of all DDC exons and exon–intron borders. However, for this patient, the results of biochemical analyses were compatible with the diagnosis of AADC deficiency: decreased CSF HVA level of 54.4 nmol/L (normal range: 97–367), decreased 5-HIAA level of 229.0 nmol/L (normal range: 236–867), and increased 3-OMD level of 809.1 nmol/L (normal level <50) in dried blood spots.

Table 1 Demographic data, mutation, and motor development of patients with AADC deficiency in Taiwan

	Sex	Termination point	First visit	Mutation 1	Mutation 2	AIMS	PDMS-2	Development
1	F	6.17	0.91	C.714+4A>T	C.714+4A>T	1	12	–
2	M	7.58	0.48	C.714+4A>T	C.714+4A>T	2	4	–
3	F	8.42	0.85	C.714+4A>T	C.714+4A>T	1	8	–
4	M	2.42	0.84	C.714+4A>T	c.1058T>C (p.L353P)	1	4	–
5	M	2.58	0.87	C.714+4A>T	C.714+4A>T	1	15	–
6	F	6.42	0.98	C.714+4A>T	c.1297dupA (p. I433Nfs*60)	2	14	–
7	M	2.58	1.98	C.714+4A>T	c.179T>C (p.V60A)	2	10	–
8[a]	F	2.83	2.72	C.714+4A>T	c.286G>A (p.G96R)	1	6	–
9	M	2.08	0.63	C.714+4A>T	C.714+4A>T	1	10	–
10	F	1.67	0.03	C.714+4A>T	C.714+4A>T	4	12	–
11	F	4.25	0.43	C.714+4A>T	C.714+4A>T	0	3	–
12	M	4.42	1.26	C.714+4A>T	C.714+4A>T	0	8	–
13	F	4.50	1.52	C.714+4A>T	C.714+4A>T	0	6	–
14	F	6.17	1.10	C.714+4A>T	c.1297dupA (p. I433Nfs*60)	0	2	–
15	M	2.00	0.00	C.714+4A>T	C.714+4A>T	3	16	–
16	F	2.67	0.31	C.714+4A>T	C.714+4A>T	1	7	–
17	M	6.58	2.42	C.714+4A>T	C.714+4A>T	4	12	–
18	F	8.25	7.31	C.714+4A>T	C.714+4A>T	5	16	–
19	M	5.79	0.75	C.714+4A>T	c.1234C>T (p.R412W)	2	11	–
20	M	4.13	3.75	C.714+4A>T	c.304G>A (p.G102S)	8	26	–
21	M	1.63	0.00	C.714+4A>T	C.714+4A>T	1	8	–
22	F	3.42	0.78	C.714+4A>T	C.714+4A>T	2	7	–
23	M	1.28	0.80	C.714+4A>T	C.714+4A>T			–
24	M	2.27	0.67	C.714+4A>T	c.1234C>T (p.R412W)			–
25	M	1.51	0.03	C.714+4A>T	C.714+4A>T			–
26	F	6.08	3.41	c.1297dupA (p. I433Nfs*60)	c.1234C>T (p.R412W)			–
27	F	5.63	2.47	C.714+4A>T	C.714+4A>T			–
28	F	4.03	1.26	C.714+4A>T	C.714+4A>T			–
29	M	7.30	1.91	c.1297dupA (p. I433Nfs*60)	c.436G>C (p.G146R)			–
30	M	6.05	0.43	C.714+4A>T	C.714+4A>T			–
31	F	3.58	3.58	C.714+4A>T	c.1297dupA (p. I433Nfs*60)			–
32	M	11.30	1.96	C.714+4A>T	c.236A>G (p.Y79C)			–
33	F	5.50	2.29	C.714+4A>T	c.179T>C (p.V60A)			–
34	F	4.39	4.39	C.714+4A>T	c.848A>C (E283A)			–
35	M	6.22	4.69	C.714+4A>T	c.58_60delTAC (p.Y20del)			–
36	M	10.62	6.71	C.714+4A>T	C.714+4A>T			–
37	M	4.08	1.63	C.714+4A>T	?			H, Sit, St

Reference sequence: NM_000790.3. c.714+4A>T mutation is also called IVS6+4A>T
– did not achieve any milestones, *H* head control, *Sit* sitting without support, *St* standing without support, *W* walking without support
[a] Ethnicity: one-half Caucasian, one-quarter Chinese, and one-quarter Thai

Growth

The body weights of patients with AADC deficiency were within normal ranges in the first few months of life (Fig. 1). Their growth began to slow down at the end of the first year, and their weight gain was minimal between 1 and 4 years of age, although all of them were treated with a combination of pyridoxine, dopamine agonists, and monoamine oxidase inhibitors. Body weight improved in three patients who survived for more than 4 years, although their weight was still below the 50th percentile. Body weight did not improve in the remaining patients, although some of them received nutrition through a nasogastric tube or gastrostomy feeding. Patient No. 37 was diagnosed at the age of 1.67 years; at that time, the patient could sit and stand but not walk. After treatment with a dopamine agonist (through the rotigotine transdermal system) and pyridoxine, the patient gained weight normally (indicated by the arrow in Fig. 1). At 6.1 years of age, the patient was able to walk freely and spoke slowly but clearly. The patient had one allele carrying the IVS6+4A>T mutation, but a mutation in the second allele was not found. The undetected mutation is likely located in the promoter, regulatory elements, or introns of the allele and is probably less harmful than the

IVS6+4A>T mutation. Patient No. 37 was the only child with AADC deficiency who developed any one of the objective motor milestones of head control, sitting ability, and standing ability.

Motor Development

With the exception of patient No. 37, all patients had profound motor deficits consistent with severe AADC deficiency (Wassenberg et al. 2017). None of these 36 patients had full head control, defined by the ability to hold their head upright in the sitting position, at their termination point in the study. None of them could sit, stand, or speak. None of these patients showed improvements in developmental milestones before their termination point in the study; that is, they did not gain any motor skills at any point during their lives.

AIMS and PDMS-2 scores were available for 22 patients at their termination points when they entered a clinical trial. Their median total raw score for the AIMS was 1 (range: 0–8), and their scores were far below the fifth percentile of normal infants aged 0–18 months (Fig. 2). Their median total raw score for the PDMS-2 was 9 (range: 2–26), and their scores were below the first percentile of normal

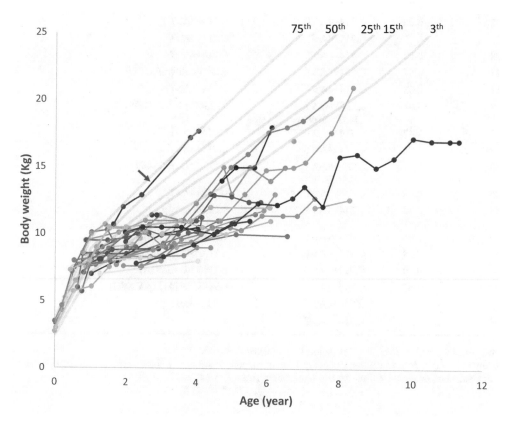

Fig. 1 Body weight of 37 patients with AADC deficiency. Body weight at each visit was plotted according to age, in comparison with the body weight distribution of normal Taiwanese female children

(Chen and Chang 2010). Each *line* represents one patient. One outlier (patient No. 37), who had significantly greater growth than other patients, is indicated by the *red arrow*

children of the same age. Their AIMS scores were strongly correlated with PDMS-2 scores [correlation coefficient (C.C.) = 0.692, $p < 0.05$, Spearman's rho test]. No correlation was observed between age and raw AIMS or PDMS-2 scores (AIMS: C.C. = 0.035, $p = 0.876$; PDMS-2: C.C. = -0.042, $p = 0.852$), because these 22 patients had virtually no gross motor development.

Discussion

In the past few years, many patients with AADC deficiency in Taiwan visited NTUH to participate in an ongoing gene therapy trial that started in 2010 (Hwu et al. 2012). A few patients were from other countries, but most of them were, at least in part, ethnically Chinese. This provided a unique opportunity to study the natural history of AADC deficiency in the Chinese population. In this study, we collected the data of a total of 37 patients, a relatively large number in one region in comparison with a global registry of 130 patients described by Wassenberg et al. (2017). In addition to the IVS6+4A>T mutation, which represented 76% of all *DDC* mutations, other recurrent mutations included c.1297dupA and p.R412W, both of which are severe mutations according to the phenotypes of patients. The allele frequency of IVS6+4A>T was found to be 0.34% in Taiwan (Chien et al. 2016). We recently saw two patients from China (who were not included in the present study); one had the genotype of homozygous IVS6+4A>T, and the other had the genotype of IVS6+4A>T/p.R412W. Because most of the Taiwanese population came from southern China, it is likely that the incidence of AADC deficiency is also high in southern China and in the Chinese population

in southeastern Asia who also came from southern China. Because of the high allele frequency of IVS6+4A>T and other severe mutations, most of our patients (36 of 37) had profound motor deficits.

Motor dysfunction is a significant component of AADC deficiency. In the present study, 36 of 37 patients did not develop full head control, sitting ability, standing ability, or speech. None of them showed improvements in these developmental milestones or gained any motor skills at any point during their lives. The study also evaluated AIMS and PDMS-2 scores that were available for 22 patients. These scores provided evidence that confirmed the lack of motor development in these patients. Typically, AIMS and PDMS-2 scores increase with age in normal children. However, the scores did not increase with age in our patients with AADC deficiency (Fig. 2). We also obtained evidence that the disease led to severe growth retardation in these patients. Regardless of disease severity, patients with AADC deficiency appeared normal at birth. However, when symptoms appeared, their growth slowed, and most of these patients ceased to gain weight after 1 year of age (Fig. 1). Motor dysfunction impaired patients' feeding and chest hygiene. Moreover, autonomic dysfunction, gastroesophageal reflux, and laryngomalacia affected the general health of these patients.

It may not be feasible to conduct controlled clinical trials for rare and rapidly fatal diseases because of the small case number and the ethical considerations involved in enrolling a placebo arm. Under such conditions, the outcome from clinical trials for rare diseases may be compared to the natural history of the diseases. Therefore, the data from the present study are critical to guide the development of treatment strategies for the disease.

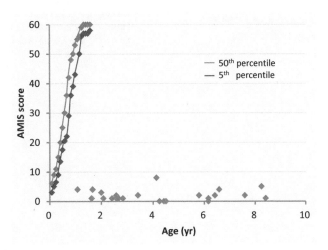

Fig. 2 AIMS scores of 22 patients with AADC deficiency. Data from patients (*blue diamond*) are depicted according to the age at the time of measurement. The *red diamonds* indicate the fifth percentile and the *green diamonds* indicate the 50th percentile of normal children (Darrah et al. 2014)

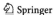

Synopsis

Patients with severe aromatic L-amino acid decarboxylase deficiency, which is more prevalent in Taiwan, present with profound motor dysfunction and failure to gain weight.

Contributions of Individual Authors

Wuh-Liang Hwu: study design, patient care, and writing.
  Yin-Hsiu Chien: patient care and writing.
  Ni-Chung Lee: patient care.
  Mei-Hsin Li: patient care assistant.

Conflict of Interest

Wuh-Liang Hwu received research grants from Agilis Biotherapeutics, USA.

Funding

Research fund for AADC deficiency, National Taiwan University Hospital.

Ethics Approval

This long-term follow-up study for AADC deficiency was approved by the Institutional Review Board of National Taiwan University Hospital (201303100RIND). All procedures followed were in accordance with the ethical standards of the responsible committee on human experimentation (institutional and national) and with the Helsinki Declaration of 1975, as revised in 2000. Informed consent was obtained from all patients before participation in the study.

References

Chen W, Chang MH (2010) New growth charts for Taiwanese children and adolescents based on World Health Organization standards and health-related physical fitness. Pediatr Neonatol 51:69–79

Chien YH, Chen PW, Lee NC et al (2016) 3-O-methyldopa levels in newborns: result of newborn screening for aromatic l-amino-acid decarboxylase deficiency. Mol Genet Metab 118:259–263

Darrah J, Bartlett D, Maguire TO, Avison WR, Lacaze-Masmonteil T (2014) Have infant gross motor abilities changed in 20 years? A re-evaluation of the Alberta Infant Motor Scale normative values. Dev Med Child Neurol 56:877–881

Graziano C, Wischmeijer A, Pippucci T et al (2015) Syndromic intellectual disability: a new phenotype caused by an aromatic amino acid decarboxylase gene (DDC) variant. Gene 559:144–148

Hwu WL, Muramatsu S, Tseng SH et al (2012) Gene therapy for aromatic L-amino acid decarboxylase deficiency. Sci Transl Med 4:134ra161

Hyland K, Clayton PT (1990) Aromatic amino acid decarboxylase deficiency in twins. J Inherit Metab Dis 13:301–304

Hyland K, Surtees RA, Rodeck C, Clayton PT (1992) Aromatic L-amino acid decarboxylase deficiency: clinical features, diagnosis, and treatment of a new inborn error of neurotransmitter amine synthesis. Neurology 42:1980–1988

Kojima K, Anzai R, Ohba C et al (2016) A female case of aromatic l-amino acid decarboxylase deficiency responsive to MAO-B inhibition. Brain and Development 38:959–963

Lee HF, Tsai CR, Chi CS, Chang TM, Lee HJ (2009) Aromatic L-amino acid decarboxylase deficiency in Taiwan. Eur J Paediatr Neurol 13:135–140

Opladen T, Cortes-Saladelafont E, Mastrangelo M et al (2016) The International Working Group on Neurotransmitter related Disorders (iNTD): a worldwide research project focused on primary and secondary neurotransmitter disorders. Mol Genet Metab Rep 9:61–66

Spitz MA, Nguyen MA, Roche S et al (2017) Chronic diarrhea in L-amino acid decarboxylase (AADC) deficiency: a prominent clinical finding among a series of ten French patients. JIMD Rep 31:85–93

Tay SK, Poh KS, Hyland K et al (2007) Unusually mild phenotype of AADC deficiency in 2 siblings. Mol Genet Metab 91:374–378

Wassenberg T, Molero-Luis M, Jeltsch K et al (2017) Consensus guideline for the diagnosis and treatment of aromatic l-amino acid decarboxylase (AADC) deficiency. Orphanet J Rare Dis 12:12

JIMD Reports
DOI 10.1007/8904_2017_56

RESEARCH REPORT

Nitisinone-Induced Keratopathy in Alkaptonuria: A Challenging Diagnosis Despite Clinical Suspicion

Andrew White · Michel C. Tchan

Received: 22 June 2017 / Revised: 23 August 2017 / Accepted: 24 August 2017 / Published online: 07 September 2017
© Society for the Study of Inborn Errors of Metabolism (SSIEM) 2017

Abstract Alkaptonuria is a rare disorder of amino acid metabolism that causes premature large joint and spine arthropathy and cardiac valvular disease. It is characterised by elevated levels of homogentisic acid. Nitisinone (NTBC) is a benzoylcyclohexane-1,3-dione that reversibly inhibits the activity of the enzymatic step immediately prior to homogentisate dioxygenase, hence reducing the production of homogentisic acid. Thus it is thought that nitisinone might be a treatment for alkaptonuria. A side effect of NTBC therapy is elevation of plasma tyrosine levels in a manner analogous to tyrosinemia type 2, another related condition which causes a painful palmoplantar hyperkeratosis and eye pathology described as conjunctivitis and herpetic-like corneal ulceration. There are only two previous reports of NTBC causing eye symptoms in patients with alkaptonuria. Here we provide further evidence of this side effect of treatment and its resolution with cessation of NTBC. Repeat challenges with NTBC provoked symptoms, but introducing a low protein diet with low dose NTBC was successful in controlling plasma tyrosine levels and the patient remained free of symptoms when levels were below 600 μmol/L. Our patient was remarkable for the low dose of NTBC that precipitated symptoms (as little as 0.5 mg daily), and for the difficulty in proving its causation despite clinical suspicion.

Introduction

Alkaptonuria is a rare disorder of amino acid metabolism that causes premature large joint and spine arthropathy and cardiac valvular disease. It is characterised by elevated levels of homogentisic acid due to autosomal recessive mutations in homogentisate dioxygenase (gene *HGD*; OMIM #203500; Phornphutkul et al. 2002), the third enzyme in the tyrosine metabolism pathway (Fig. 1). Homogentisic acid is further metabolised to benzoquinone acetic acid which forms a melanin-like polymer and is deposited in the connective tissue (a process known as ochronosis), leading to the major disease manifestations as well as characteristic dark discolouration of the earlobes, irises and nail beds.

Nitisinone (NTBC) is a benzoylcyclohexane-1,3-dione that reversibly inhibits the activity of the enzymatic step immediately prior to homogentisate dioxygenase, thus reducing the production of homogentisic acid. Thus it is thought that NTBC might be a treatment for alkaptonuria (Introne et al. 2011). NTBC has been used for many years in the treatment of hereditary tyrosinemia type 1, a related disorder with a metabolic block further down the tyrosine metabolism pathway at fumarylacetoacetase. A side effect of NTBC therapy is elevation of plasma tyrosine levels in a manner analogous to tyrosinemia type 2 (due to deficiency of tyrosine transaminase), a related condition which causes a painful palmoplantar hyperkeratosis and eye pathology described as conjunctivitis and herpetic-like corneal ulcera-

Communicated by: Daniela Karall

A. White · M.C. Tchan
Westmead Hospital, Westmead, NSW, Australia

A. White · M.C. Tchan
Sydney University, Sydney Medical School, Westmead, NSW, Australia

M.C. Tchan (✉)
Department of Genetic Medicine, Westmead Hospital, PO Box 533, Wentworthville, NSW 2145, Australia
e-mail: Michel.tchan@health.nsw.gov.au

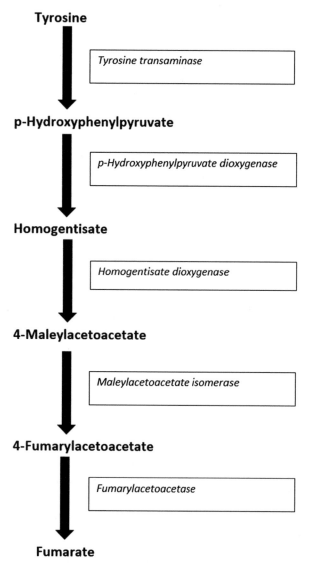

Tyrosine

Tyrosine transaminase

p-Hydroxyphenylpyruvate

p-Hydroxyphenylpyruvate dioxygenase

Homogentisate

Homogentisate dioxygenase

4-Maleylacetoacetate

Maleylacetoacetate isomerase

4-Fumarylacetoacetate

Fumarylacetoacetase

Fumarate

Fig. 1 Tyrosine metabolism pathway

tion. There are only two previous reports of NTBC causing eye symptoms in patients with alkaptonuria (Introne et al. 2011; Stewart et al. 2014); here we provide further evidence of this side effect of treatment and its resolution with cessation of NTBC.

Case Description

The patient, AA, is a 21-year-old female whose diagnosis of alkaptonuria had been made when she was 5 years old. She was commenced on vitamin C from the ages of 7 until 15 years and was maintained on a mildly restricted protein diet from 13 years. Evaluation at age 21 documented an unremarkable history, with no symptoms of major joint arthropathy, and normal psychomotor development. Physical examination was likewise unremarkable (height 162 cm

and weight 52 kg), and echocardiography and plain X-rays were reported as normal. Prior to NTBC therapy, the level of urinary homogentisic acid was 1,066 mmol/mol creatinine (<0.2 mmol/mol creatinine) and plasma tyrosine was 37 μmol/L (32–114 μmol/L).

She was commenced on low dose NTBC (0.5 mg daily), and noted mild eye discomfort and occasional visual blurring 4 days later. Optometry review did not detect any abnormalities other than mild hypermetropia; her symptoms of occasional visual blurring and eye discomfort continued without increasing in severity. At 4 months of therapy the homogentisic acid level was 249 mmol/mol creatinine; tyrosine was not measured. The dose of NTBC was increased after 7 months to 1.5 mg daily. At 10 months of treatment, she noted significantly increased eye irritation, inflammation and photophobia. The level of homogentisic acid was 47.7 mmol/mol creatinine and tyrosine was 760 μmol/L. Optometry review noted corneal irritation and photosensitivity without corneal crystalline deposits or keratopathy, and antibiotics were prescribed for a presumed bacterial infection. She was advised to cease NTBC. Symptoms did not improve over 3 days and urgent ophthalmology review diagnosed blepharitis for which steroids were prescribed. Symptoms settled over 1 week and NTBC was recommenced. Symptoms rapidly recurred and repeat ophthalmology examination finally revealed corneal crystalline deposits (Fig. 2). Symptoms and tyrosine crystals resolved within days of cessation of NTBC.

A subsequent challenge with NTBC at 1 mg daily invoked mild symptoms 4 weeks after commencement, and crystals were again seen. NTBC was ceased for 2 weeks with resolution of symptoms. A further trial of NTBC at 0.5 mg daily, with natural dietary protein restricted to 40 g, supplemented with 15 g protein equivalent of tyrosine-free supplement, has resulted in plasma tyrosine levels ranging from 285 to 625 μmol/L. Over this period of 4 months the patient was almost symptom free. Mild ocular irritation which resolved without intervention over 3 days was noted by the patient around the time that plasma tyrosine level was 625 μmol/L. The subsequent tyrosine level was 461 μmol/L.

Discussion

Is there causation between tyrosine levels and ophthalmic pathology in NTBC-treated alkaptonuria? Our data from this single case report does not provide a definitive answer to this question; however, high tyrosine levels (760 μmol/L) correlated with worse symptoms in our patient. Experience in tyrosinemia type II is instructive here, as untreated patients may have levels over 1,000 μmol/L, and dietary management (low protein diet with appropriate formula supplementation) lowers levels to under 600 μmol/L with

a

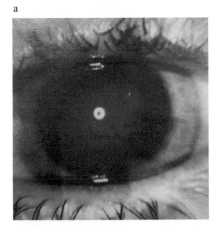

b

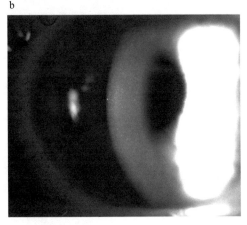

Fig. 2 Images taken at 10 months after commencing NTBC. Plasma tyrosine level was 760 µmol/L. (a) Keratopathy. (b) Tyrosine crystalline deposits

doses – 2 mg daily and 2 mg on alternate days (Introne et al. 2011; Stewart et al. 2014).

This case demonstrates that subjective clinical symptoms from crystalline keratopathy may be found in the absence of crystals being seen, and at tyrosine levels elevated by relatively low doses of NTBC. We suggest that plasma tyrosine levels be monitored after first commencing NTBC, and maintained at levels of <600 µmol/L with a combination of tailored NTBC dosage and dietary management. We also suggest that ophthalmology review be instituted at first clinical ophthalmology symptoms, and consideration of NTBC dose reduction or cessation be undertaken regardless of whether signs of keratopathy are seen.

Synopsis

NTBC used for the treatment of alkaptonuria may cause corneal crystalline keratopathy at low doses, and symptoms may be apparent prior to ophthalmic changes.

Declaration of Competing/Conflicts of Interest

The authors declare that they have no conflicts of interest.

References

Introne WJ, Perry MB, Troendle J et al (2011) A 3-year randomized therapeutic trial of nitisinone in alkaptonuria. Mol Genet Metab 103(4):307–314

Phornphutkul C, Introne WJ, Perry MB et al (2002) Natural history of alkaptonuria. N Engl J Med 347(26):2111–2121

Ranganath LR, Milan AM, Hughes AT et al (2016) Suitability Of Nitisinone In Alkaptonuria 1 (SONIA 1): an international, multicentre, randomised, open-label, no-treatment controlled, parallel group, dose-response study to investigate the effect of once daily nitisinone on 24-h urinary homogentisic acid excretion in patients with alkaptonuria after 4 weeks of treatment. Ann Rheum Dis 75(2):362–367

Scott CR (2006) The genetic tyrosinemias. Am J Med Genet Part C Semin Med Genet 142C:121–126

Stewart RM, Briggs MC, Jarvis JC, Gallagher JA, Ranganath L (2014) Reversible keratopathy due to hypertyrosinaemia following intermittent low-dose nitisinone in alkaptonuria: a case report. JIMD Rep 17:1–6

resolution of ophthalmic symptoms within days to weeks (Scott 2006).

The particular sensitivity of our patient to NTBC was surprising. Doses of 10 mg daily are being used in the SONIA-2 trial, and doses of up to 8 mg daily were tolerated in the SONIA-1 trial (Ranganath et al. 2016). Two other patients known to the authors have not had symptoms despite being on higher doses than this patient (up to 2 mg daily), and with plasma tyrosine levels of up to 800 µmol/L. It is worth noting, however, that the two previously described cases of nitisinone-induced keratopathy in alkaptonuria occurred in patients receiving relatively low

JIMD Reports
DOI 10.1007/8904_2017_53

RESEARCH REPORT

ALG13-CDG with Infantile Spasms in a Male Patient Due to a De Novo *ALG13* Gene Mutation

Wienke H. Galama ·
Sandra L.J. Verhaagen – van den Akker ·
Dirk J. Lefeber · Ilse Feenstra · Aad Verrips

Received: 24 March 2017 / Revised: 20 July 2017 / Accepted: 28 July 2017 / Published online: 09 September 2017
© Society for the Study of Inborn Errors of Metabolism (SSIEM) 2017

Abstract A boy presented at the age of 3.5 months with a developmental delay. He developed infantile spasms with hypsarrhytmia on EEG 1 month later. Additional symptoms were delayed visual development, asymmetrical hearing loss, hypotonia, and choreoathetoid movements. He also had some dysmorphic features and was vulnerable for infections. He was treated successively with vigabatrin, prednisolone, valproic acid, nitrazepam, and lamotrigine without a lasting clinical effect, but showed a treatment response to levetiracetam. Cerebral MRI showed hypoplasia of the corpus callosum and a mild delay in myelination. Further investigations including metabolic screening and glycosylation studies by transferrin isoelectric focusing were all considered to be normal. Whole-exome sequencing identified a de novo mutation in the *ALG13* gene (c.320A>G, p.(Asn107Ser)). Mutations in this gene, which is located on the X-chromosome, are associated with congenital disorders of glycosylation type I (CDG-I). Mass spectrometric analysis of transferrin showed minor glycosylation abnormalities. The c.320A>G mutation in *ALG13* has until now only been described in girls and was thought to be lethal for boys. All girls with this specific mutation presented with a similar phenotype of developmental delay and severe early onset epilepsy. In two girls glycosylation studies were performed which showed a normal glycosylation pattern. This is the first boy presenting with an epileptic encephalopathy caused by the c.320A>G mutation in the *ALG13* gene. Since glycosylation studies are near-normal in patients with this mutation, the diagnosis of ALG13-CDG can be missed if genetic studies are not performed.

Introduction

Infantile spasms is the most common early-onset epileptic encephalopathy (EOEE). The outcome can be poor and includes developmental delay and chronic refractory epilepsy in 70% of cases. Prognosis depends on the underlying etiology, which is diverse and includes infections, perinatal events, and genetic disorders (Michaud et al. 2014).

The underlying etiology is unknown in about 40% of patients with infantile spasms, once called "idiopathic" cases. Nowadays, it is assumed that genetic factors play an important role in these patients (Osborne et al. 2010; Berg and Scheffer 2011). However, in only a small proportion a particular monogenetic defect has been identified (Dimassi et al. 2016; Møller et al. 2016; Michaud et al. 2014). A specific epilepsy syndrome can be caused by mutations in different genes, but at the same time the same gene and even same mutation can lead to broad phenotypic variations (Møller et al. 2016; Berg and Scheffer 2011). De novo mutations seem to play an important role in sporadic patients with infantile spasms. Genomic analyses, such as whole-exome sequencing (WES), can help to identify causative genes and significantly improve the diagnostic

Communicated by: Eva Morava, MD PhD

W.H. Galama (✉) · S.L.J. Verhaagen – van den Akker · A. Verrips
Department of Neurology/Pediatric Neurology, Canisius Wilhelmina Hospital, Nijmegen, The Netherlands
e-mail: w.galama@cwz.nl

D.J. Lefeber
Department of Neurology, Translational Metabolic Laboratory, Radboud University Medical Centre, Nijmegen, The Netherlands

I. Feenstra
Department of Human Genetics, Radboud University Medical Centre, Nijmegen, The Netherlands

yield (Helbig et al. 2016; Allen et al. 2013; Michaud et al. 2014). In several studies a family-based WES approach is used to reveal the underlying genetic cause in patients with an unexplained intellectual disability or epileptic encephalopathy. After sequencing the exomes of the patient and unaffected parents, the exome of the patient can be analyzed for mutations in genes involved in autosomal recessive and X-linked inheritance, but also for de novo mutations by excluding inherited variants (de Ligt et al. 2012; Allen et al. 2013).

Previous reports implicated a role of *ALG13* mutations in the etiology of epileptic encephalopathies (Myers et al. 2016; Smith-Packard et al. 2015; Allen et al. 2013; Dimassi et al. 2016; Michaud et al. 2014; Hino-Fukuyo et al. 2015; Kobayashi et al. 2016). Particularly, the c.320A>G mutation in *ALG13* has been identified several times in girls with infantile spasms. *ALG13* gene mutations were also described as a cause of X-linked intellectual disability and congenital disorders of glycosylation type I (ALG13-CDG) (Bissar-Tadmouri et al. 2014; de Ligt et al. 2012; Timal et al. 2012). The *ALG13* gene is located on the X-chromosome and encodes a protein that heterodimerizes with ALG14 to form a complex in the endoplasmic reticulum that catalyzes the second step of protein N-glycosylation (Averbeck et al. 2008). This multistep process is identical for each N-glycosylated protein and is important for the structure and function of these glycoproteins. Genetic defects in this process cause CDG-I, with a highly variable multisystem phenotype. The diagnostic test for almost all N-linked CDG-I-subtypes is serum transferrin isoelectric focusing (IEF) (Sparks and Krasnewich 2005). However, there are CDG-I-subtypes with a normal transferrin profile, such as ALG13-CDG and ALG14-CDG, which expresses the need for additional glycoprotein biomarkers. With advanced mass spectrometry it is possible to analyze released glycans from serum proteins and perform intact glycoprotein analysis, which provides quantitative glycan structural information. Until now, advanced mass spectrometry has mostly been used in research settings. But since it is a quick test with high sensitivity and specificity the added value of mass spectrometry in the diagnostic process is increasingly recognized (Van Scherpenzeel et al. 2016). For most CDG-I-subtypes the defective enzyme is known, but enzymatic assays have not yet been developed or are scarcely available for most (Sparks and Krasnewich 2005). Also the clinical phenotypes of CDG-I-subtypes are not discriminative. Therefore, genetic testing can be helpful to define the specific CDG-I-subtype (Timal et al. 2012).

Here, we present a boy with infantile spasms and near-normal glycosylation studies. WES identified a c.320A>G mutation in *ALG13*, which has previously only been described in girls.

Case Report

A 3.5 months old boy was referred with delayed motor development. Before, he had been admitted to the hospital twice for recurrent infections. Parents had noticed at the age of 6 weeks that he did not make eye contact or smile yet. Apart from a delay in motor development with axial hypotonia, a plagiocephaly, mild retrognathia, mild torticollis, and scoliosis with a hemivertebra L1–L2 were present. Furthermore, asymmetrical hearing loss of 60–70 dB with an underdeveloped right auricle was detected. At the age of 4.5 months he presented with infantile spasms and hypsarrhythmia on EEG.

Cerebral MRI showed hypoplasia of the corpus callosum and a mild delay in myelination. Genetic and metabolic screening at the age of 3.5 months, including glycosylation studies by transferrin isoelectric focusing, were considered to be normal. Mass spectrometric analysis of transferrin revealed a lack of one glycan of ~6%, while a repeat plasma sample at the age of 15 months revealed a lack of one glycan of ~8% (in controls <4%). A family-based WES in the proband and parents was performed, revealing a de novo c.320A>G mutation (p.(Asn107Ser)) in the *ALG13* gene, confirming the diagnosis ALG13-CDG.

Treatment with vigabatrin was started, with addition of nitrazepam. Because of a lack of treatment response after 2 weeks, the vigabatrin was withdrawn, and high dose prednisolone (10 mg four times daily) was started, leading to a cessation of seizures and disappearance of hypsarrhythmia on EEG within 2 weeks. Two weeks later prednisolone was decreased slowly and valproic acid was started. At that time, generalized choreatiform movements were noted. A few weeks later he presented with generalized tonic-clonic seizures, occurring during an upper respiratory tract infection. Lamotrigine was added, but did not result in a cessation of seizure activity and was withdrawn. Recently, levetiracetam was started which resulted in a reduction of seizure activity for several weeks up to now.

Discussion

The infantile spasms and developmental delay in our patient are due to ALG13-CDG caused by a de novo c.320A>G mutation in the *ALG13* gene, resulting in the substitution of serine for asparagine at position 107 in the ALG13 protein (p.(Asn107Ser)). This de novo mutation is the most frequently described *ALG13* mutation, leading to a developmental delay and epileptic encephalopathy. It has so far only been described in 12 girls in a heterozygous state, but never in a male patient (de Ligt et al. 2012; Allen et al. 2013; Michaud et al. 2014; Smith-Packard et al. 2015;

Dimassi et al. 2016; Kobayashi et al. 2016; Myers et al. 2016; Wong 2016). Previously, it was even assumed that this variant caused embryonic lethality in males because only female patients were reported (Smith-Packard et al. 2015).

It is unclear by which mechanism the c.320A>G variant in *ALG13* is acting. Haploinsufficiency, causing the loss of one functional *ALG13* copy, could have been the case in girls with this mutation. However, one would expect that it would cause a more severe phenotype or even lethality in boys because of the hemizygous state. Therefore, a dominant negative effect as mechanism of action seems more likely in this *ALG13* variant. In girls this would lead not only to the loss of one normal functioning *ALG13* copy, but also to a dysfunction of the remaining copy resulting in even less or no residual function. This could lead to a more or less similar phenotype in both male and female patients.

In two girls with the c.320A>G mutation in the *ALG13* gene, serum transferrin isoelectric focusing was performed and showed a normal glycosylation pattern. In one girl mass spectrometric analysis was also performed, which was normal as well (Smith-Packard et al. 2015). It is unclear if mass spectrometry was performed in the second girl (Dimassi et al. 2016). In our patient analysis of glycosylation by transferrin isoelectric focusing was normal, but a slightly reduced glycosylation with a lack of one glycan was demonstrated by mass spectrometry. In a patient with a different *ALG13* mutation (c.280A>G; p.(Lys94Glu)), transferrin isoelectric focusing revealed clearly increased asialo- and disialotransferrin fractions, in agreement with a CDG-I (Timal et al. 2012). Given that positions 1–125 of the *ALG13* gene are related to glycosyltransferase activity, one would expect that both mutations would lead to a defect in glycosylation and thus a clearly abnormal glycosylation pattern (Uniprot 2017). Since glycosylation studies are near-normal in patients with the c.320A>G mutation in *ALG13*, the diagnosis of ALG-13 CDG can be missed if genetic studies are not performed.

Because most *ALG13* mutations were identified with WES in patient cohorts with either epileptic encephalopathies or intellectual disability, there is only limited data available on the clinical spectrum caused by *ALG13* mutations and outcome of these patients.

Nearly all girls described with the c.320A>G mutation were normal at birth, but developed early onset seizures and a severely delayed development or even developmental regression after a few months. One case showed a developmental delay since birth (de Ligt et al. 2012). Most patients presented initially with infantile spasms. Later on they developed more polymorphic seizures, such as myoclonic-tonic spasms, focal seizures, or generalized epilepsy. Vigabatrin did not improve infantile spasms in one patient (Michaud et al. 2014), and even worsened the additional movement disorder in another (Myers et al. 2016). In about half of the patients, the infantile spasms initially responded to ACTH treatment (Allen et al. 2013; Michaud et al. 2014; Smith-Packard et al. 2015; Hino-Fukuyo et al. 2015). However, during follow-up the majority regained epileptic seizures, which sometimes responded to antiepileptic drugs (such as topiramate) or a ketogenic diet, and were refractory in others (Allen et al. 2013; Michaud et al. 2014; Smith-Packard et al. 2015; Kobayashi et al. 2016; Myers et al. 2016).

As in our case, some patients with a mutation in *ALG13* had an extrapyramidal movement disorder such as dyskinesias or choreoathetoid movements (Myers et al. 2016; Kobayashi et al. 2016; Timal et al. 2012), whereas also dysmorphic features were reported (de Ligt et al. 2012; Dimassi et al. 2016). Furthermore, visual development may be affected by a defect of the *ALG13* gene, since it has been described in almost half of the cases (our report, Timal et al. 2012; de Ligt et al. 2012; Allen et al. 2013; Smith-Packard et al. 2015; Dimassi et al. 2016; Hino-Fukuyo et al. 2015).

Other *ALG13* variants have been described previously in males (Table 1). In most of these cases, the mutation was maternally inherited. Timal et al. described the first male patient with ALG13-CDG, due to a de novo c.280A>G mutation in the *ALG13* gene, who died at the age of 1 year. He presented with refractory epilepsy with polymorphic seizures, multiple congenital anomalies, bilateral optic nerve atrophy, recurrent infections, increased bleeding tendency, as well as extrapyramidal and pyramidal signs. His glycosylation pattern suggested a CDG-I. No structural abnormalities were found by assaying lipid-linked oligosaccharides (LLO) synthesis, neither was a clear deficiency shown by indirect analysis of the GlcNAc transferase activities. Direct assaying of ALG13/ALG14 enzyme activity was necessary to detect a functional deficit in glycosylation and confirm the diagnosis of ALG13-CDG. Unfortunately this assay is not available anymore at this moment. Since this entire analysis is a lengthy biochemical process and the clinical phenotypes of CDG-I-subtypes are not discriminative, the authors recommend the use of next generation sequencing techniques to diagnose CDG-I-subtypes like ALG13-CDG (Timal et al. 2012).

Another boy initially had a normal motor development until the age of 4 months. Then he developed bilateral optic atrophy with nystagmus and lack of visual fixation. Subsequently, infantile spasms appeared with hypsarrhythmia on EEG. A missense mutation of *ALG13* (c.880C>T) was detected. He inherited this variant from his mother who was an asymptomatic carrier. No glycosylation studies were reported (Hino-Fukuyo et al. 2015).

In a third boy with Lennox-Gastaut syndrome, a c.1641A>T mutation in *ALG13* was identified. Both his mother and grandmother were asymptomatic carriers. No

Table 1 Summary of male patients with *ALG13* mutation

	Age onset epilepsy	Sex	ALG13 variant	Inheritance	Protein change	Clinical findings	MRI	Glycosylation studies	Response to treatment
This report	4.5 months	M	c.320 A>G	De novo	p.(Asn107Ser)	Developmental delay, infantile spasms/polymorphic seizures, hypotonia, dysmorphic features, delayed visual maturation, choreatiform movements	Hypoplasia corpus callosum and mild delay myelination	Transferrin IEF normal. Mass spectrometry lack of one glycan (~6–8% ref: <4%)	Spasms initially responded to prednisolone. No effect of vigabatrin, nitrazepam, and valproic acid. Response to levetiracetam
Timal et al. (2012)	Not reported	M	c.280A>G Hemizygous	De novo	p.(Lys94Glu)	Seizures, microcephaly, delayed visual maturation, extrapyramidal/pyramidal signs, hepatomegaly, bleeding tendency, swelling hand/feet/eyelids	Not reported	N-glycosylation defect type I (ALG13-CDG)	Refractory polymorphic epilepsy, died at age of 1 year
Bissar-Tadmouri et al. (2014)	Not applicable	M (n = 4)	c.3221A>G Hemizygous	Maternal inheritance	p.(Tyr1074Cys)	Intellectual disability	Normal	Not tested	Not applicable
Hino-Fukuyo et al. (2015)	5 months	M	c.880C>T Hemizygous	Maternal inheritance	p.(Pro294Ser)	Developmental delay, infantile spasms/seizures, delayed visual maturation	Anomaly corpus callosum	Not reported	Spasms responded to pyridoxine and ACTH, followed by tonic/myoclonic seizures responding to AED
Møller et al. (2016)	Not reported	M	c.1641A>T	Maternal inheritance	p.(Gln547His)	Lennox-Gastaut syndrome	Not reported	Not reported	Not reported

further information about this case was provided (Møller et al. 2016).

Finally, an *ALG13* missense mutation (c.3221A>G) was discovered in four male siblings with X-linked intellectual disability. Their mother was an asymptomatic carrier of the mutation as well. No epileptic seizures or other neurological symptoms were described in these boys, and glycosylation studies were not mentioned (Bissar-Tadmouri et al. 2014).

In conclusion, the c.320A>G mutation in the *ALG13* gene may not only cause ALG13-CDG with a severe early onset epileptic encephalopathy and developmental delay in girls, but can also be the cause of this phenotype in boys. Glycosylation studies in these patients are near-normal, which means that the diagnosis of ALG13-CDG can be missed if genetic studies are not performed (Myers et al. 2016; Smith-Packard et al. 2015; Allen et al. 2013; Dimassi et al. 2016; Michaud et al. 2014; Kobayashi et al. 2016).

Synopsis

The c.320A>G mutation in *ALG13*, which until now has only been described in girls, can also be a cause of ALG13-CDG with near-normal glycosylation studies in boys.

Author Contributions

Wienke H. Galama: Conception and design, literature review, drafted article, coordination of revisions, guarantor.

Sandra L. J. Verhaagen – van den Akker: Provided clinical data and drafted case report.

Dirk J. Lefeber: Provided glycosylation data, contribution of intellectual content and critical revision.

Ilse Feenstra: Provided genetic data, contribution of intellectual content and critical revision.

Aad Verrips: Conception and design, provided clinical data, contribution of intellectual content and critical revision.

Corresponding author: Wienke H. Galama.

Compliance with Ethics Guidelines

Conflict of Interest

Wienke Galama declares that she has no conflict of interest.

Sandra Verhaagen – van den Akker declares that she has no conflict of interest.

Dirk Lefeber declares that he has no conflict of interest.

Ilse Feenstra declares that she has no conflict of interest.

Aad Verrips declares that he has no conflict of interest.

Informed Consent

All procedures followed were in accordance with the ethical standards of the responsible committee on human experimentation (institutional and national) and with the Helsinki Declaration of 1975, as revised in 2000. Informed consent was obtained from all patients for being included in the study. Additional informed consent was obtained from all patients for which identifying information is included in this article.

Funding

The authors confirm independence from sponsors.

References

Allen AS, Berkovic SF, Cossette P et al (2013) De novo mutations in epileptic encephalopathies. Nature 501:217–221

Averbeck N, Gao XD, Nishimura S, Moller DN (2008) Alg13p, the catalytic subunit of the endoplasmic reticulum UDP-GlcNAc glycosyltransferase, is a target for proteasomal degradation. Mol Biol Cell 19:2169–2178

Berg AT, Scheffer IE (2011) New concepts in classification of the epilepsies: entering the 21st century. Epilepsia 52:1058–1062

Bissar-Tadmouri N, Donahue WL, Al-Gazali L, Nelson SF, Bayrak-Toydemir P, Kantarci S (2014) X chromosome exome sequencing reveals a novel ALG13 mutation in a nonsyndromic intellectual disability family with multiple affected male siblings. Am J Med Genet A 164A:164–169

de Ligt J, Willemsen MH, van Bon BW et al (2012) Diagnostic exome sequencing in persons with severe intellectual disability. N Engl J Med 367:1921–1929

Dimassi S, Labalme A, Ville D et al (2016) Whole-exome sequencing improves the diagnosis yield in sporadic infantile spasm syndrome. Clin Genet 89:198–204

Helbig KL, Farwell Hagman KD, Shinde DN et al (2016) Diagnostic exome sequencing provides a molecular diagnosis for a significant proportion of patients with epilepsy. Genet Med 18:898–905

Hino-Fukuyo N, Kikuchi A, Arai-Ichinoi N et al (2015) Genomic analysis identifies candidate pathogenic variants in 9 of 18 patients with unexplained West syndrome. Hum Genet 134(6):649–658

Kobayashi Y, Tohyama J, Kato M et al (2016) High prevalence of genetic alterations in early-onset epileptic encephalopathies associated with infantile movement disorders. Brain and Development 38:285–292

Michaud JL, Lachance M, Hamdan FF et al (2014) The genetic landscape of infantile spasms. Hum Mol Genet 23:4846–4858

Møller RS, Larsen LH, Johannesen KM et al (2016) Gene panel testing in epileptic encephalopathies and familial epilepsies. Mol Syndromol 7:210–219

Myers CT, McMahon JM, Schneider AL et al (2016) De novo mutations in SLC1A2 and CACNA1A are important causes of epileptic encephalopathies. Am J Hum Genet 99:287–298

Osborne JP, Lux AL, Edwards SW et al (2010) The underlying etiology of infantile spasms (West syndrome): information from the United Kingdom Infantile Spasms Study (UKISS) on contemporary causes and their classification. Epilepsia 51:2168–2174

Smith-Packard B, Myers SM, Williams MS (2015) Girls with seizures due to the c.320A>G variant in ALG13 do not show abnormal glycosylation pattern on standard testing. JIMD Rep 22:95–98

Sparks SE, Krasnewich DM (2005) Congenital disorders of N-linked glycosylation and multiple pathway overview. In: GeneReviews [Internet]. University of Washington, Seattle, Seattle. Updated 12 Jan 2017

Timal S, Hoischen A, Lehle L et al (2012) Gene identification in the congenital disorders of glycosylation type I by whole-exome sequencing. Hum Mol Genet 21:4151–4161

Uniprot (2017) UniProtKB – Q9NP73 (ALG13_HUMAN). http://www.uniprot.org/uniprot/Q9NP73#family_and_domains

Van Scherpenzeel M, Willems E, Lefeber DJ (2016) Clinical diagnostics and therapy monitoring in the congenital disorders of glycosylation. Glycoconj J 33:345–358

Wong S (2016) ALG13: X-linked gene causes severe neurological disease in females. http://blog.courtagen.com/alg13-x-linked-gene-causes-severe-neurological-disease-in-females

JIMD Reports
DOI 10.1007/8904_2017_55

RESEARCH REPORT

Liver Failure as the Presentation of Ornithine Transcarbamylase Deficiency in a 13-Month-Old Female

Farrah Rajabi · Lance H. Rodan · Maureen M. Jonas ·
Janet S. Soul · Nicole J. Ullrich · Ann Wessel ·
Susan E. Waisbren · Wen-Hann Tan · Gerard T. Berry

Received: 02 June 2017 / Revised: 16 August 2017 / Accepted: 18 August 2017 / Published online: 09 September 2017
© Society for the Study of Inborn Errors of Metabolism (SSIEM) 2017

Abstract Ornithine transcarbamylase deficiency (OTCD) is an X-linked urea cycle disorder with variable expressivity in heterozygous females. While liver function testing is often abnormal in patients with OTCD, liver failure is uncommon on presentation. A 13-month-old female with no significant past medical history presented with irritability, right arm weakness, and decreased appetite. Initial workup revealed hepatic dysfunction with an INR of 3.4, ammonia level of 75 μmol/L, and abnormal brain MRI with gyral edema with restricted diffusion, and patchy signal abnormality in basal ganglia. The MRI findings led to a putative diagnosis of acute disseminated encephalomyelitis prompting corticosteroid treatment. As steroid treatment was begun, she developed significant hepatocellular dysfunction with ALT 2,222 U/L, AST 630 U/L, prolonged INR, and elevated ammonia (213 μmol/L). Neurologic signs resolved and her ammonia level decreased (43 μmol/L) without further intervention; however, she had ongoing acute liver failure with coagulopathy and episodic irritability, managed as seronegative autoimmune hepatitis with partial response to corticosteroid therapy. At 18 months of age she presented with severe irritability with markedly increased ammonia (417 μmol/L).

Plasma amino acids obtained several days prior to this acute episode demonstrated elevation in glutamine (2,725 μmol/L) and alanine (1,459 μmol/L). Biochemical testing demonstrated elevation of urine orotic acid (>240.6 mmol/mol creatinine). Genetic testing confirmed a heterozygous nonsense mutation in the *OTC* gene (c.958C>T, R320X). After treatment with ammonia scavengers and a protein-restricted diet, hepatic function normalized and irritability resolved. The diagnosis of a urea cycle disorder should be considered in patients with unexplained hepatic dysfunction.

Communicated by: Johannes Häberle

F. Rajabi · L.H. Rodan · A. Wessel · S.E. Waisbren · W.-H. Tan ·
G.T. Berry (✉)
Division of Genetics and Genomics, Boston Children's Hospital,
300 Longwood Ave, Boston, MA 02115, USA
e-mail: Gerard.Berry@childrens.harvard.edu

M.M. Jonas
Division of Gastroenterology, Hepatology, and Nutrition,
Boston Children's Hospital, Boston, MA 02115, USA

J.S. Soul · N.J. Ullrich
Department of Neurology, Boston Children's Hospital, Boston, MA
02115, USA

Introduction

Ornithine transcarbamylase (OTC) deficiency (OTCD) is an X-linked urea cycle disorder that affects both males and females (Brusilow and Horwich 2014). OTCD is caused by mutations in the gene encoding OTC on chromosome Xp11, and it is the most frequent urea cycle disorder (Tuchman et al. 2008). The urea cycle disorders have overlapping presentations that are primarily the consequence of hyperammonemia, including vomiting, lethargy, progressive somnolence, irritability, agitation, disorientation, and ataxia; however, the age of presentation and prognosis can vary from fatality in the neonatal period to variable severity appearing any time thereafter (Brusilow and Horwich 2014). Variable clinical expressivity can be marked in individuals with residual OTC enzyme activity, particularly heterozygous females (Batshaw et al. 1986). Late presentations in childhood may be associated with weaning from breast milk to higher protein formula or cow's milk, high-protein meals, or catabolism related to infection (Brusilow and Horwich 2014).

OTCD may be suspected based on an elevated blood ammonia concentration, elevated serum glutamine concentration, low serum citrulline concentration, and elevated urine orotic acid; a definitive diagnosis is based on the identification of a pathogenic variant in the *OTC* gene, a pedigree analysis, elevated baseline urinary orotic acid level or after an allopurinol challenge test, and/or reduced OTC enzyme activity in liver or intestinal tissue (Tuchman et al. 2008). OTC enzyme activity has low sensitivity for diagnosis in female patients because of the X-chromosome inactivation pattern (Yorifuji et al. 1998). Liver involvement is increasingly recognized as a common complication of OTCD, which is present in more than 50% of patients presenting with symptomatic OTCD (Gallagher et al. 2014; Laemmle et al. 2016). The pathophysiology of the liver dysfunction in OTCD is poorly understood, and primary hepatic presentations are uncommonly reported.

Clinical Report

A 13-month-old female with no significant past medical history presented with irritability, right arm weakness, and decreased appetite. The report of her newborn screening was normal, and amino acid details were unknown. Her parents were healthy and the family history was negative for metabolic disorders, other than a maternal history of hypothyroidism. There was, however, a strong history of autoimmune disorders, including scleroderma in the paternal grandmother, Crohn's disease, rheumatoid arthritis, and colitis in the paternal cousins, and hypothyroidism and alopecia in the maternal aunts. Initial workup revealed significant hepatic dysfunction with an INR of 3.4, plasma ammonia level of 75 μmol/L, and abnormal brain MRI with gyral edema of both hemispheres with restricted diffusion, and patchy signal abnormality in basal ganglia with diffusion abnormality (Fig. 1). Differential diagnoses at

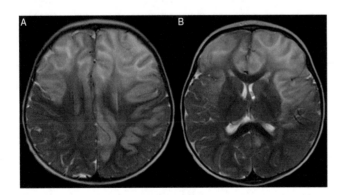

Fig. 1 Axial T2 brain MRI on initial presentation at 13 months old demonstrated increased T2 signal intensity (**a**, **b**) throughout the frontal hemispheres extending posteriorly without enhancement or restricted diffusion (not shown)

the time of initial presentation included cytomegalovirus infection, metabolic disorder, autoimmune hepatitis, and acute disseminated encephalomyelitis (ADEM). The MRI findings led to a putative diagnosis of ADEM, which prompted treatment with high dose intravenous corticosteroids. Shortly after steroid treatment was initiated, she was found to have significant hepatic dysfunction with ALT 2,222 U/L, AST 630 U/L, prolonged INR (3.4), and elevated plasma ammonia (213 μmol/L). Metabolic studies performed 4 days after her initial presentation included a plasma amino acid quantitation of glutamine (1,248 μmol/L; reference range 303–1,459), alanine (691 μmol/L; reference range 119–523), and citrulline (15 μmol/L; reference range 4–50). Apparently, since the glutamine and citrulline levels were within the reference range at an outside laboratory facility, these values were not investigated further. Additionally, as the plasma sample had to be sent out to another outside facility, the results were not returned until 3 weeks after the initial presentation. A urine organic acid analysis was also performed yielding elevations in lactate, 3-hydroxybutyrate, acetoacetate, 4-hydroxyphenyllactate, and 4-hydroxyphenylpyruvate.

Neurologic symptoms resolved and her ammonia level decreased (55 μmol/L) with intravenous fluids with 10% glucose and intralipids, but she continued to have ongoing acute liver failure with coagulopathy as her INR was >1.5, but without hyperbilirubinemia. Her liver dysfunction was managed as seronegative autoimmune hepatitis demonstrating partial response to corticosteroid therapy. Liver biopsy revealed mild lymphocytic inflammation with focal mild ballooning of hepatocytes. She had episodic irritability that correlated with episodes of aminotransferase elevations, though ammonia levels were not measured with these episodes.

At 18 months of age, she had a subacute presentation of severe irritability with decreased speech, and was found to have markedly increased ammonia on admission (443 μmol/L). Her family had noted unusual odors and recrudescence of her right-sided weakness for several days prior to presentation. Plasma amino acids obtained 3 days prior to this acute episode demonstrated marked elevation in glutamine (2,725 μmol/L) and alanine (1,459 μmol/L). These amino acids also demonstrated a citrulline level of 15 μmol/L (reference range 3–45 μmol/L) and arginine level of 30 μmol/L (reference range 29–116 μmol/L). She was admitted for treatment of hyperammonemia and further metabolic diagnostic evaluation for possible urea cycle disorder. The hyperammonemia resolved after treatment with ammonia scavengers and a protein-restricted diet supplemented with essential amino acids and increased calories. Brain MRI demonstrated diffuse parenchymal volume loss (Fig. 2). Hepatic function gradually normalized (Figs. 3 and 4) and irritability resolved.

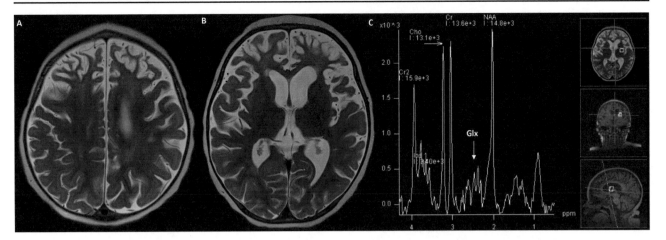

Fig. 2 Axial T2 brain MRI at 18 months old (**a**, **b**) demonstrated interval increase in abnormal white matter T2 prolongation in frontal lobes, parietal lobes, posterior temporal lobes, and centrum semiovale as well as diffuse parenchymal volume loss. MR spectroscopy (**c**) with a glutamine–glutamate (Glx) complex peak

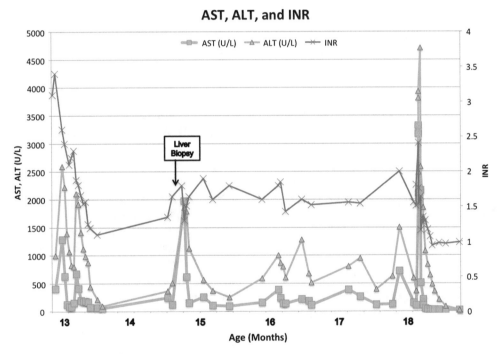

Fig. 3 Laboratory trends from time of initial presentation at 13 months old. Reference ranges AST 2–40 mmol/L, ALT 3–30 mmol/L; INR 0.87–1.13

Biochemical testing demonstrated marked elevation of urine orotic acid (>240.6 mmol/mol creatinine). Genetic testing confirmed a heterozygous nonsense pathogenic variant in the *OTC* gene (c.958C>T, R320X) (Demmer et al. 1996; Kim et al. 2006; Caldovic et al. 2015). This known pathogenic variant is predicted to eliminate the protein through nonsense-mediated mRNA decay. The same mutation was originally identified in a symptomatic Korean female patient with several male relatives who had died of presumptive OTCD (Yoo et al. 1996). Maternal testing for the R320X variant was negative.

On follow up at 20 months of age, she was making good developmental progress. Assessment with the Bayley Scales of Infant and Toddler Development (Third Edition) showed cognitive abilities within the average range, although she was mildly delayed in all areas. On the Bayley Cognitive Index, she attained a composite score of 85, with skills at approximately a 17-month level. On the Language Composite scale, she received a composite score of 89, with skills at the 16-month level in receptive communication and at the 19-month level in expressive communication. On the Bayley Motor Composite, she

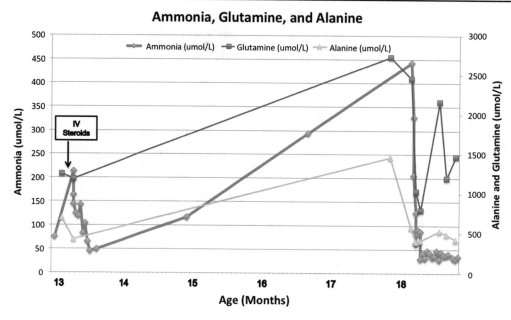

Fig. 4 Laboratory trends from time of initial presentation at 13 months old. Reference ranges ammonia 50–80 mmol/L; glutamine 427–907 mmol/L, alanine 122–578 mmol/L

received a score of 73, with gross motor skills at the 14-month level and fine motor skills at the 12-month level. At 3 years and 4 months of age, assessment with the Wechsler Preschool and Primary Scale of Intelligence (Fourth Edition) composite scores showed average cognitive abilities (scores 85–115 represent average). Her composite score for full scale IQ was 109 with a verbal comprehension score of 114, a visual spatial score of 112, and a working memory score of 87.

Discussion

The variable clinical expressivity of male and female OTCD patients can make diagnosis challenging. Although liver failure is a known complication of OTCD, acute liver failure as the initial presentation of OTCD is uncommon, with a few reports in the medical literature presenting as young as 14 months old (Mustafa and Clarke 2006; Mira and Boles 2012). Liver involvement is present in more than half of the patients who present with symptomatic OTCD. In a historical cohort study of 49 patients with symptomatic OTCD at two centers in the United States with symptomatic OTC, 29% met criteria for acute liver failure, and three patients presented with acute liver failure (Gallagher et al. 2014). In another study cohort of Swiss patients with OTCD, 6 of 15 symptomatic female patients were found to have acute liver failure which was recurrent in 2 patients, and 6 of 9 male patients had acute liver failure (Laemmle et al. 2016).

The pathogenesis of liver injury in OTCD is unknown. Liver biopsy in previous cases has demonstrated acute hepatocellular injury with mild lobular necrosis (Gallagher et al. 2014). Reports of hepatocellular carcinoma in some patients with OTCD and other urea cycle disorders have raised concern that urea cycle disorders increase the risk of liver cancer due to chronic liver damage by toxic metabolites, and perhaps to the toxicity of excess carbamoyl phosphate, which leads to either high energy phosphate toxicity or to diversion into the pyrimidine synthesis pathway, resulting in dysregulation of the nucleotide pool (Wilson et al. 2012). In the recent report from Laemmle et al. the authors hypothesized that ammonia toxicity contributes directly to the development of acute liver failure by impairing hepatic protein synthesis with in vitro studies of hepatocytes from unaffected donors. The cell culture studies demonstrated reduced production rate of albumin upon ammonium chloride (NH_4Cl) treatment, and a moderate increase of AST indicating a negative effect of ammonia on mitochondrial integrity (Laemmle et al. 2016). Our patient's treatment with steroids may have precipitated her crisis with hyperammonemia (Gascon-Bayarri et al. 2015; Lipskind et al. 2011).

Our patient's initial presentation with right-arm weakness was also unusual. Acute focal neurologic deficits are atypical in urea cycle disorders, but have been described in urea cycle disorders with neurologic symptoms occurring both with and without acute hyperammonemia (Keegan et al. 2003). Keegan et al. presented a 6-year-old male with partial OTCD who presented with ataxia and dysarthria that resolved after treatment. In a review of neurologic outcomes of 28 patients with OTCD, 7 patients had long-term neurologic involvement on examination; 2 with spastic quadriparesis, 4 with mixed dystonic/spastic hemiplegia, and 1 with spastic diplegia (Nicolaides et al. 2002).

The diagnosis of a urea cycle disorder should be considered in patients with unexplained hepatic dysfunction. Older infants may even present with liver failure. Under these circumstances, any patient who has had an appropriate but unsuccessful medical evaluation for common etiologies of liver failure should undergo a systematic metabolic investigation including measurement of plasma amino acid levels. Ongoing unexplained hepatic dysfunction should prompt consideration of genetic evaluation for urea cycle disorders. Recognition of a urea cycle disorder as a component of the differential diagnosis can prompt early metabolic workup and diagnosis to initiate specific lifesaving metabolic treatment. Elevated glutamine associated with an increased waste nitrogen burden may precede clinical symptoms of hyperammonemia (Brusilow and Horwich 2014). The increase in glutamine and alanine associated with hyperammonemia can be an important diagnostic clue since elevation in these amino acids may precede hyperammonemia and the onset of clinical signs and symptoms.

Synopsis

Urea cycle disorders can present with hepatic failure, and early recognition of a urea cycle disorder in the differential of hepatic dysfunction can prompt early metabolic diagnosis to initiate specific lifesaving metabolic treatment.

Contributions of Individual Authors

Farrah Rajabi drafted the initial manuscript and approved the final manuscript as submitted.

Lance H. Rodan and Gerard T. Berry assisted in drafting, and revised the manuscript and approved the final manuscript as submitted.

Maureen M. Jonas, Janet Soul, Nicole J. Ullrich, Ann Wessel, Susan E. Waisbren, and Wen-Hann Tan reviewed and revised the manuscript and approved the final manuscript as submitted.

Compliance with Ethics Guidelines

Farrah Rajabi, Lance Rodan, Maureen M. Jonas, Janet Soul, Nicole J. Ullrich, Ann Wessel, Susan E. Waisbren,

Wen-Hann Tan, and Gerard T. Berry declare that they have no conflict of interest.

This is a descriptive report, and all patient information has been anonymized to ensure patients are not identifiable. All patients have provided informed consent to genetic testing. This chapter does not contain any studies with human or animal subjects performed by any of the authors.

References

Batshaw ML, Msall M, Beaudet AL, Trojak J (1986) Risk of serious illness in heterozygotes for ornithine transcarbamylase deficiency. J Pediatr 108:236–241

Brusilow SW, Horwich AL (2014) Urea cycle enzymes. In: Valle D, Beaudet AL, Vogelstein B, Kinzler KW, Antonarakis SE, Ballabio A, Gibson K, Mitchell G (eds) The online metabolic and molecular bases of inherited disease. McGraw-Hill, New York

Caldovic L, Abdikarim I, Narain S, Tuchman M, Morizono H (2015) Genotype-phenotype correlations in ornithine transcarbamylase deficiency: a mutation update. J Genet Genomics 42:181–194

Demmer LA, Kim JM, de Martinville B, Dowton SB (1996) A novel missense mutation in the exon containing the putative ornithine-binding domain of the OTC enzyme in a female. Hum Mutat 7:279

Gallagher RC, Lam C, Wong D, Cederbaum S, Sokol RJ (2014) Significant hepatic involvement in patients with ornithine transcarbamylase deficiency. J Pediatr 164:720–725.e6

Gascon-Bayarri J, Campdelacreu J, Estela J, Rene R (2015) Severe hyperammonemia in late-onset ornithine transcarbamylase deficiency triggered by steroid administration. Case Rep Neurol Med 2015:453752

Keegan CE, Martin DM, Quint DJ, Gorski JL (2003) Acute extrapyramidal syndrome in mild ornithine transcarbamylase deficiency: metabolic stroke involving the caudate and putamen without metabolic decompensation. Eur J Pediatr 162:259–263

Kim G-H, Choi J-H, Lee H-H, Park S, Kim S-S, Yoo H-W (2006) Identification of novel mutations in the human ornithine transcarbamylase (OTC) gene of Korean patients with OTC deficiency and transient expression of the mutant proteins in vitro. Hum Mutat 27:1159

Laemmle A, Gallagher RC, Keogh A, Stricker T, Gautschi M, Nuoffer J-M, Baumgartner MR, Häberle J (2016) Frequency and pathophysiology of acute liver failure in ornithine transcarbamylase deficiency (OTCD). PLoS One 11:e0153358

Lipskind S, Loanzon S, Simi E, Ouyang D (2011) Hyperammonemic coma in an ornithine transcarbamylase mutation carrier following antepartum corticosteroids. J Perinatol 31:682–684

Mira V, Boles RG (2012) Liver failure with coagulopathy, hyperammonemia and cyclic vomiting in a toddler revealed to have combined heterozygosity for genes involved with ornithine transcarbamylase deficiency and Wilson disease. JIMD Rep 3:1–3

Mustafa A, Clarke JTR (2006) Ornithine transcarbamoylase deficiency presenting with acute liver failure. J Inherit Metab Dis 29:586

Nicolaides P, Liebsch D, Dale N, Leonard J, Surtees R (2002) Neurological outcome of patients with ornithine carbamoyltransferase deficiency. Arch Dis Child 86:54–56

Tuchman M, Lee B, Lichter-Konecki U, Summar ML, Yudkoff M, Cederbaum SD, Kerr DS, Diaz GA, Seashore MR, Lee H-S, McCarter RJ, Krischer JP, Batshaw ML (2008) Cross-sectional multicenter study of patients with urea cycle disorders in the United States. Mol Genet Metab 94:397–402

Wilson JM, Shchelochkov OA, Gallagher RC, Batshaw ML (2012) Hepatocellular carcinoma in a research subject with ornithine transcarbamylase deficiency. Mol Genet Metab 105:263–265

Yoo HW, Kim GH, Lee DH (1996) Identification of new mutations in the ornithine transcarbamylase (OTC) gene in Korean families. J Inherit Metab Dis 19:31–42

Yorifuji T, Muroi J, Uematsu A, Tanaka K, Kiwaki K, Endo F, Matsuda I, Nagasaka H, Furusho K (1998) X-inactivation pattern in the liver of a manifesting female with ornithine transcarbamylase (OTC) deficiency. Clin Genet 54:349–353

JIMD Reports
DOI 10.1007/8904_2017_60

RESEARCH REPORT

The Use of d2 and Benton Tests for Assessment of Attention Deficits and Visual Memory in Teenagers with Phenylketonuria

Bozena Didycz · Magdalena Nitecka ·
Miroslaw Bik-Multanowski

Received: 24 July 2017 / Revised: 24 August 2017 / Accepted: 01 September 2017 / Published online: 24 September 2017
© Society for the Study of Inborn Errors of Metabolism (SSIEM) 2017

Abstract Hyperphenylalaninemia-related, subtle deficits of attention and of working memory are often reported in adolescents with phenylketonuria. Focused neuropsychological tests can be used to detect such deficits and to confirm the presence of poor metabolic control in the periods between routine blood phenylalanine tests, which are rarely performed in many patients from this age group due to their low treatment adherence.

We assessed the practical value of the d2 test of attention and of the Benton visual retention test for identification of teenagers, who have a high risk of brain dysfunction due to hyperphenylalaninemia. We analyzed the correlation between neuropsychological test scores achieved by 30 patients and their blood phenylalanine profiles since the neonatal period.

We observed strong correlation between the Concentration Performance scores on the d2 test and the quality of metabolic control within last month prior to the follow-up visit in the outpatient clinic ($r = -0.72$; $p = 0.0003$). The mean z-score was significantly higher in patients with good metabolic control than in those with poorly controlled hyperphenylalaninemia (0.44 vs. -1.12; $p = 0.00002$). On contrary, the results of the Benton visual retention test did not correlate significantly with the individual blood phenylalanine profiles.

We believe that neuropsychological assessment should be used in adolescents with phenylketonuria on a regular basis in order to increase the self-awareness in these patients and, consequently, to increase their treatment adherence and safety. The d2 test can be effectively used for detection of attention deficits and seems to be a valuable supplementary procedure for routine follow-up.

Abbreviations
Phe Phenylalanine
PKU Phenylketonuria
SD   Standard deviation

Introduction

Phenylketonuria (PKU, OMIM 261600) is the most common inborn error of metabolism in man. If untreated, the disease manifests as severe brain damage resulting from chronic hyperphenylalaninemia. Treatment using a low-phenylalanine diet should start in the neonatal period (ideally before the tenth day of life) and should be continued for the rest of the patient's life. If properly treated, patients usually show normal development (Blau et al. 2010) although discrete neuropsychological abnormalities have also been reported (Enns et al. 2010).

Metabolic control is usually sufficient in prepubertal patients. Unfortunately, adolescents with PKU typically relax the dietary regimen, resulting in insufficient treatment adherence (Walter et al. 2002). Poorly controlled hyperphenylalaninemia often leads to high brain phenylalanine concentrations, with a resulting imbalance in production of neurotransmitters and eventually dysmyelination (Feillet et al. 2010). Neuropsychological deficits are often observed

Communicated by: Avihu Boneh, MD, PhD, FRACP

B. Didycz · M. Bik-Multanowski (✉)
Department of Medical Genetics, Faculty of Medicine, Jagiellonian University Medical College, Kraków, Poland
e-mail: miroslaw.bik-multanowski@uj.edu.pl

M. Nitecka
Department of Developmental and Clinical Psychology, University Children's Hospital, Kraków, Poland

🌀 Springer

in teenagers and adults without proper metabolic control of hyperphenylalaninemia. These include typical deficits in executive function, attention problems, and decreased working memory (Feillet et al. 2010; Bik-Multanowski et al. 2011).

Current guidelines for PKU include frequent monitoring of blood phenylalanine (Phe) concentration with subsequent adjustment of the dietary treatment if blood levels exceed the maximal recommended range (0.36 mmol/L in patients younger than 12 and 0.6 mmol/L thereafter). In addition, the cognitive status should be assessed twice, at approximately 12 and 18 years of age (van Spronsen et al. 2017). However, other than the classic Wechsler Intelligence Tests, no specific methods for cognitive assessment are recommended. Previous studies show that overall intelligence in PKU patients correlates with the extent of life-long hyperphenylalaninemia (Waisbren et al. 2007). Thus, the sporadic use of Wechsler tests has little practical value for early detection and quantitative measurement of PKU-specific cognitive impairment. The use of focused tests that allow assessment of subtle neuropsychological deficits (e.g., in the areas of attention and working memory) could increase the chance for early detection of the above deficits and, consequently, for timely adjustment of the patient's dietary therapeutic regimen. Therefore, establishment of a robust set of neuropsychological tests, suitable for repeated assessment of teenagers with PKU would be useful.

In our previous paper, we reported using the computerized Cambridge Neuropsychological Test Automated Battery (CANTAB) tests to measure attention span and working memory in patients with PKU (Bik-Multanowski et al. 2011). Here, we evaluate the practical value of two similar, classic paper-and-pencil tests: the d2 test of attention and the Benton visual retention test.

Material and Methods

A group of 30 PKU patients who were treated early and continuously, aged 13–18 years and with normal intellectual development, participated in the study. All patients had been followed up in our clinic since infancy, and dietary treatment was initiated in their first month of life. Table 1 presents details on the studied population, including the treatment initiation time and IQ results at study entry.

Study participants took the d2 test of attention and the Benton visual retention test. In the d2 test the individual examined is asked to cross out any letter "d" with two marks above it or below it in any order. The surrounding distractors are usually similar to the target stimulus, for example a "p" with two marks or a "d" with one or three marks (Semrud-Clikeman and Teeter Ellison 2009; Leclercq and Zimmermann 2002).

Six parameters of the d2 test were assessed: total number of items processed (TN), raw score of errors (E), percentage of errors (E%), total number of items minus error scores (TN-E), the fluctuation rate (FR), and concentration performance (CP; the number of correct d2 items minus commission errors). The performance of the above-listed measures was referenced to normative data to control for the effect of age (Dajek and Brickenkamp 2010).

In the Benton test, the person examined is shown ten designs one at a time and asked to reproduce each one as exactly as possible on plain paper from memory (Benton 1992).

One parameter was assessed with regard to the Benton visual retention test: the number error score. The type A method of test administration was used (viewing each design for 10 s before reproducing them).

We analyzed 5,378 results of blood phenylalanine concentration to evaluate the influence of the most recent and historical Phe fluctuations on the attention capacity and visual working memory in teenagers with PKU. Correlations of the test results with the medium- and long-term blood Phe dynamics were analyzed to assess the usefulness of the d2 and the Benton tests in assessing the quality of metabolic control in PKU patients.

The one-sided Pearson's correlation statistic was used and Sidak's correction for multiple comparisons was applied to calculate the statistical significance of the correlation coefficient, r. The level of $r = 0.52$ was considered significant (corrected $p < 0.003$; $N = 30$; number of comparisons $= 42$). Student's t-test was used for comparison of test scores between patients with good and insufficient metabolic control.

The local ethics committee approved the study and the patients provided informed consent for participation.

Results

Only three out of six parameters assessed in the d2 test significantly correlated with blood Phe levels (TN, TN-E, and CP). The strongest correlations were observed for the period 1 month prior to neuropsychological testing. However, the highest values of the r coefficient were noted for the CP value ($r = -0.72$). The mean z-score for CP was significantly higher in patients with good metabolic control (0.44 vs. -1.12; $p = 0.00002$ in t-test). The correlation between neuropsychological score and blood phenylalanine concentration was weaker for longer observational periods (1 year, 2 years, first 12 years of life) and for the life-long changeability of Phe (standard deviation of Phe values in the first 12 years of life). The details on neuropsychological examinations and Phe dynamics are presented in Table 2.

Table 1 The PKU patients

Patient	Gender	Treatment start (day of life)	Age at psychological assessment (years)	IQ (Wechsler scale)	Mutations of the *PAH* gene
1	F	31	14	93	p.R408W/p.R408W
2	M	26	13	124	p.R408W/p.R408W
3	F	27	13	110	p.R408W/p.R408W
4	F	12	13	123	p.R408W/p.R408W
5	M	20	14	115	p.R408W/p.R243Q
6	F	31	15	113	p.R408W/p.I283F
7	F	13	15	99	p.[T63P;H64N]/N
8	F	11	13	141	p.R408W/p.R408W
9	M	28	17	96	p.R408W/p.R408W
10	F	20	15	132	p.R408W/N
11	F	19	14	97	p.R408W/p.R408W
12	F	16	14	116	p.R408W/N
13	M	10	18	117	p.R408W/p.R408W
14	F	8	12	124	p.R408W/p.R408W
15	F	19	13	106	p.R408W/p.R408W
16	M	11	14	112	p.R408W/p.R408W
17	F	13	12	107	p.R408W/p.E183Q
18	F	9	14	119	p.R408W/p.R408W
19	M	11	12	122	p.R408W/p.R408W
20	F	13	14	87	p.R408W/p.I283F
21	F	14	17	105	p.R408W/p.I283F
22	M	13	15	110	p.R408W/IVS2+5G>C
23	F	10	14	107	p.R408W/p.R408W
24	M	27	15	101	p.R408W/p.R408W
25	M	14	14	122	p.R408W/IVS9-2C>A
26	F	31	18	90	p.R408W/p.R408W
27	F	29	14	108	p.R408W/p.R408W
28	F	14	17	106	p.R408W/p.R408W
29	F	27	14	107	p.R408W/p.R243X
30	M	14	15	104	p.R408W/p.R408W

N not identified

Figure 1 shows the relationship between CP and the mean blood Phe concentrations during a period of 1 month before neuropsychological testing. The average CP decreases below the 50th percentile in patients in whom blood Phe exceeds approximately 0.6 mmol/L (10 mg/dL).

In contrast to the d2 test of attention, the results of the Benton visual retention test did not correlate significantly with the assessed Phe values.

Table 3 presents details of the statistical analysis.

Discussion

In our study, we assessed the practical value of two classic neuropsychological tests to assess the treatment effectiveness in adolescents with PKU. Our results show that the extent of hyperphenylalaninemia exerts mainly short-term and medium-term effects on the neuropsychological capacity of teenage patients in the field of attention. This is consistent with previous findings in patients with phenylketonuria (Schmidt et al. 1996) and it may correspond with the postulated effect of fluctuations in dopamine concentration in the prefrontal cortex because of brain tyrosine deficits secondary to hyperphenylalaninemia (De Groot et al. 2010). The neurotransmitter-related prefrontal cortex dysfunction in patients with phenylketonuria seems to be largely reversible, in contrast to dysmyelination, which was reported after several years of poor metabolic control in PKU patients.

The frequency of blood phenylalanine monitoring, which is high in young children, becomes low and

Table 2 Blood phenylalanine (Phe) and the results of neuropsychological tests

	The d2 test of attention (z-score)						Benton test Number error score (sten)	Mean Phe prior to neuropsychological assessment (mmol/L)				
Patient	TN	E	E%	TN − E	FR	CP		Last month	Last year	Last 2 years	First 12 years of life	Standard deviation in first 12 years
1	1.75	−0.55	0	1.55	1.03	1.64	6	0.16	0.29	0.22	0.31	0.24
2	1.12	−0.70	−0.22	1.12	0.20	1.55	5	0.19	0.29	0.25	0.28	0.24
3	0.91	−0.80	−0.33	0.87	1.64	0.52	NA	0.24	0.45	0.53	0.47	0.47
4	−0.95	−1.55	0.25	−0.95	1.40	−0.49	7	0.32	0.5	0.49	0.35	0.14
5	−0.25	0.67	1.12	−0.1	0.91	0.1	7	0.36	0.37	0.41	0.32	0.38
6	−0.27	−0.12	0.25	−0.12	1.22	−0.07	6	0.37	0.31	0.28	0.49	0.33
7	0.17	−0.25	0	0.33	1.75	0.12	6	0.39	0.22	0.16	0.32	0.24
8	0.84	0.17	0.73	1.12	0.64	1.22	6	0.4	0.4	0.42	0.3	0.27
9	−0.1	0.49	0.61	0.07	1.64	0.12	10	0.52	0.51	0.49	0.64	0.33
10	1.75	−1.40	−1.34	1.40	0.91	−0.15	4	0.58	0.63	0.59	0.42	0.26
11	−0.33	0.61	1.12	−0.12	−0.35	0.07	10	0.6	0.35	0.29	0.41	0.3
12	0.22	1.88	2.32	0.35	1.64	0.61	5	0.6	0.55	0.53	0.43	0.26
13	−2.32	1.28	1.12	−1.88	0.91	−1.28	6	0.62	0.49	0.5	0.49	0.31
14	−0.67	0.77	1.12	−0.67	−0.30	−0.30	NA	0.7	0.67	0.61	0.69	0.52
15	0.52	−0.80	−0.84	−0.49	−0.38	0.05	6	0.73	0.88	0.83	0.63	0.42
16	−0.15	−1.08	−1.17	−0.46	1.28	−1.34	6	0.73	0.64	0.64	0.7	0.38
17	1.03	−0.22	0.20	1.08	0.52	−2.32	6	0.8	1.02	0.71	0.46	0.41
18	−0.64	0.49	0.55	−0.33	2.32	−0.33	4	0.85	0.77	0.73	0.68	0.24
19	−0.27	0.33	0.25	−0.1	−0.30	0.15	7	0.9	1.1	0.97	0.49	0.36
20	0.41	−0.27	−0.02	0.46	0.12	0.35	7	0.94	0.91	0.86	0.46	0.31
21	−0.91	0.05	0.25	−0.84	−0.07	−0.35	6	0.98	0.53	0.56	0.39	0.32
22	−1.03	−1.08	−1.34	−1.55	0.44	−2.32	5	1.0	1.01	0.92	0.45	0.28
23	−1.40	0.49	0.25	−1.34	0.91	−1.03	6	1.06	1.21	1.12	0.52	0.27
24	−0.35	0.61	0.61	−0.22	2.32	0.02	5	1.07	0.91	0.8	0.65	0.33
25	−1.88	−0.74	−1.22	−2.05	0.25	−2.32	5	1.13	1.02	0.79	0.52	0.38
26	−1.55	−0.52	−0.67	−1.75	1.28	−1.64	6	1.13	0.82	0.64	0.34	0.26
27	0.15	−1.34	−1.40	−0.30	1.03	−1.64	5	1.18	1.14	1.07	0.61	0.49
28	−1.88	0.05	−0.22	−1.75	−0.07	−1.88	6	1.19	1.14	1.07	0.41	0.26
29	−1.40	−0.61	−1.17	−1.75	0.77	−1.75	6	1.31	0.86	0.86	0.76	0.38
30	−0.70	−1.28	−1.75	−1.75	0.05	−2.32	4	1.37	1.3	0.73	0.7	0.33

NA not assessed

insufficient in many teenagers with PKU because of low treatment adherence (Walter et al. 2002). Thus, measurement of Phe concentration might be not adequate to assess short-term metabolic control. In our study, analysis of the d2 test of attention scores revealed a strong inverse correlation of hyperphenylalaninemia and concentration performance in teenagers with PKU. Assessment of this parameter could be helpful in monitoring the quality of metabolic control in the last period preceding the follow-up visit at a metabolic clinic. However, repeated use of the d2 test of attention requires further study to determine if it consistently reflects treatment effectiveness, especially because of the possible learning effect in tested individuals. Other tests, such as computerized tests, e.g. CANTAB or Amsterdam Neuropsychological Tasks (Bik-Multanowski et al. 2011; De Sonneville 1999), could be used alternately with classic paper-and-pencil methods. It should also be noted that a baseline level of attention should be measured in every patient to enable further monitoring of concentration performance. We believe that such complex neuropsy-

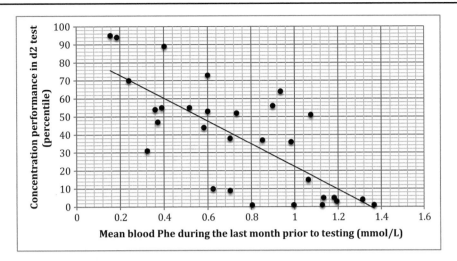

Fig. 1 The relationship between concentration performance and blood phenylalanine

chological assessments could be routinely performed at 12 years of age, as was recently suggested (van Spronsen et al. 2017), and then could be repeated every 1–2 years.

In addition, careful analysis of Fig. 1 leads to conclusions supporting the current recommendations on maintenance of blood phenylalanine below 0.6 mmol/L in patients over 12 years of age. Hyperphenylalaninemia exceeding this threshold can result in worsening concentration performance.

Interestingly, the mean IQ score in our patients was relatively high. The learning effect (most of the participants of this study were assessed with use of the same version of the WISC-R test in primary school), or the so-called Flynn effect, referring to "ageing" of the test, which can result in overestimation of IQ scores in a population over time (Flynn 1987), could explain this finding.

In conclusion, we believe that assessment of attention using the d2 test in teenagers with PKU can be a valuable supplement to the standard biochemical monitoring of PKU treatment effectiveness. In our opinion the d2 test can be helpful in selection of those teenagers with PKU, who underperform at school due to attention deficits and who could increase their cognitive potential in case of intensification of the every-day dietary, psychological, and social support.

Take-Home Message

The d2 test, a classic neuropsychological paper-and-pencil diagnostic tool, can be used for assessment of dynamics of attention deficits, which are typically observed in patients with phenylketonuria.

Corresponding Author (the Guarantor of the Article)

Prof. Miroslaw Bik-Multanowski, MD, PhD, Department of Medical Genetics, ul. Wielicka 265, 30-336 Kraków, Poland; e-mail: miroslaw.bik-multanowski@uj.edu.pl.

Compliance with Ethics Guidelines

Conflict of Interest

Bozena Didycz, Magdalena Nitecka and Miroslaw Bik-Multanowski declare that they have no conflict of interest.

Informed Consent

All procedures followed were in accordance with the ethical standards of the responsible committee on human experimentation (institutional and national) and with the Helsinki Declaration of 1975, as revised in 2000 (5). Informed consent was obtained from all patients for being included in the study.

Contributions of Individual Authors

BD designed the study, collected and analyzed data, and wrote the manuscript, MN performed the psychological tests, contributed to data analysis and consulted the manuscript, MBM helped to design and supervised the study, consulted and partially modified the methodology, contributed to data analysis and to drafting of the manuscript.

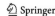

Table 3 Statistical analysis of the results

	The tests used in the study						The Benton visual retention test (sten)
	The d2 test of attention (z-score)						
The assessed periods	TN (total number of items processed)	E (raw score of errors)	$E\%$ (percentage of errors)	TN − E (total number of items − error score)	FR (the fluctuation rate)	CP (concentration performance)	Number error score
Correlations between the results of neuropsychological tests and blood phenylalanine parameters (Pearson correlation)							
Mean Phe in the last month before tests	$r = -\mathbf{0.58}$, $p = \mathbf{0.028}$	$r = -0.09$	$r = -0.42$	$r = -\mathbf{0.66}$, $p = \mathbf{0.003}$	$r = -0.3$	$r = -\mathbf{0.72}$, $p = \mathbf{0.0003}$	−0.28
Mean Phe 1 year before tests	$r = -0.41$	$r = -0.18$	$r = -0.47$	$r = -0.51$	$r = -0.37$	$r = -\mathbf{0.61}$, $p = \mathbf{0.01}$	−0.32
Mean Phe 2 years before tests	$r = -0.38$	$r = -0.1$	$r = -0.38$	$r = -0.46$	$r = -0.31$	$r = -0.56$	−0.25
Mean of yearly Phe means (first 12 years of life)	$r = -0.29$	$r = -0.01$	$r = -0.23$	$r = -0.37$	$r = -0.05$	$r = -0.44$	−0.12
Standard deviation of Phe (first 12 years of life)	$r = 0.03$	$r = -0.01$	$r = -0.14$	$r = -0.01$	$r = -0.29$	$r = -0.1$	−0.02
Mean results of neuropsychological tests vs. metabolic control in the last month before psychological assessment							
Patients with Phe within the recommended limit (0.6 mmol/L)	0.40	−0.13	0.38	0.46	1.05	0.44	6.55
Patients with Phe above the recommended limit	−0.72	−0.21	−0.3	−0.87	0.62	−1.12	5.65
Comparison of both groups (t-test)	$p = \mathbf{0.002}$	$p = 0.8$	$p = 0.06$	$p = \mathbf{0.0002}$	$p = 0.11$	$p = \mathbf{0.00002}$	$p = 0.17$

Statistically significant values are presented in bold

Ethics Approval

The study was approved by the regional Ethics Committee (29/KBL/OIL/2011).

Funding

This work was supported by the Nutricia Research Foundation (grant number 02/2011).

References

Benton AL (1992) Benton visual retention test, 5th edn. Psychological Corporation, San Antonio

Bik-Multanowski M, Pietrzyk JJ, Mozrzymas R (2011) Routine use of CANTAB system for detection of neuropsychological deficits in patients with PKU. Mol Genet Metab 102:210–213

Blau N, van Spronsen FJ, Levy HL (2010) Phenylketonuria. Lancet 376:1417–1427

Dajek ER, Brickenkamp R (2010) Polska standaryzacja Testu d2, testu badania uwagi R. Brickenkampa. ERDA, Warsaw

De Groot MJ, Hoeksma M, Blau N, Reijngoud DJ, van Spronsen FJ (2010) Pathogenesis of cognitive dysfunction in phenylketonuria: review of hypotheses. Mol Genet Metab 99:S86–S89

De Sonneville LMJ (1999) Amsterdam neuropsychological tasks: a computer-aided assessment program. In: Brinker BPLM, Beek PJ, Brand AN, Maarse SJ, Mulder LJM (eds) Computers in psychology: cognitive ergonomics, clinical assessment and computer-assisted learning. Swets & Zeitlinger, Lisse, pp 187–203

Enns GM, Koch R, Brumm V, Blakely E, Suter R, Jurecki E (2010) Suboptimal outcomes in patients with PKU treated early with diet alone: revisiting the evidence. Mol Genet Metab 101:99–109

Feillet F, van Spronsen FJ, MacDonald A et al (2010) Challenges and pitfalls in the management of phenylketonuria. Pediatrics 126:333–341

Flynn JR (1987) Massive IQ gains in 14 nations: what IQ tests really measure. Psychol Bull 101:171–191

Leclercq M, Zimmermann P (2002) Applied neuropsychology of attention: theory, diagnosis and rehabilitation. Psychology Press, Hove, p 193

Schmidt E, Burgard P, Rupp A (1996) Effects of concurrent phenylalanine levels on sustained attention and calculation speed in patients treated early for phenylketonuria. Eur J Pediatr 155: S82–S86

Semrud-Clikeman M, Teeter Ellison PA (2009) Child neuropsychology: assessment and interventions for neurodevelopmental disorders, 2nd edn. Springer, Berlin, p 111

van Spronsen FJ, van Wegberg AM, Ahring K et al (2017) Key European guidelines for the diagnosis and management of patients with phenylketonuria. Lancet Diabetes Endocrinol 5 (9):743–756

Waisbren S, Noel K, Fahrbach K et al (2007) Phenylalanine blood levels and clinical outcomes in phenylketonuria: a systematic literature review and meta-analysis. Mol Genet Metab 92:63–70

Walter JH, White FJ, MacDonald A (2002) How practical are recommendations for dietary control in phenylketonuria? Lancet 360:55–57

JIMD Reports
DOI 10.1007/8904_2017_62

Asymptomatic Corneal Keratopathy Secondary to Hypertyrosinaemia Following Low Dose Nitisinone and a Literature Review of Tyrosine Keratopathy in Alkaptonuria

M. Khedr · S. Judd · M. C. Briggs · A. T. Hughes ·
A. M. Milan · R. M. K. Stewart · E. A. Lock ·
J. A. Gallagher · L. R. Ranganath

Received: 18 May 2017 / Revised: 17 August 2017 / Accepted: 04 September 2017 / Published online: 24 September 2017
© Society for the Study of Inborn Errors of Metabolism (SSIEM) 2017

Abstract Nitisinone, although unapproved for use in alkaptonuria (AKU), is currently the only homogentisic acid lowering therapy with a potential to modify disease progression in AKU. Therefore, safe use of nitisinone off-label requires identifying and managing tyrosine keratopathy. A 22-year-old male with AKU commenced 2 mg daily nitisinone after full assessment. He was issued an alert card explaining potential ocular symptoms such as red eye, tearing, ocular pain and visual impairment and how to manage them. On his first and second annual follow-up visits to the National Alkaptonuria Centre (NAC), there was no corneal keratopathy on slit lamp examination. On his third follow-up annual visit to the NAC, he was found to have typical dendritiform corneal keratopathy in both eyes which was asymptomatic. Nitisinone was suspended until a repeat slit lamp examination, 2 weeks later, confirmed that the keratopathy had resolved. He recommenced nitisinone 2 mg daily with a stricter low protein diet. On his fourth annual follow-up visit to the NAC, a routine slit lamp examination showed mild corneal keratopathy in the left eye. This is despite him reporting no ocular symptoms. This case highlights the fact that corneal keratopathy can occur without symptoms and any monitoring plan with off-label use of nitisinone in AKU will need to take this possibility into account. This is also the first time that typical corneal keratopathy has been described with the use of low dose nitisinone in AKU without symptoms.

Communicated by: Pascale de Lonlay

M. Khedr (✉) · A.T. Hughes · A.M. Milan · L.R. Ranganath
Department of Clinical Biochemistry and Metabolic Medicine,
Liverpool Clinical Laboratories, Royal Liverpool University Hospital,
Prescot Street, Liverpool L7 8XP, UK
e-mail: mkhedr@liverpool.ac.uk

S. Judd
Department of Nutrition and Dietetics, Royal Liverpool University
Hospital, Prescot Street, Liverpool L7 8XP, UK

M.C. Briggs
Department of Ophthalmology, Royal Liverpool University Hospital,
Prescot Street, Liverpool L7 8XP, UK

A.T. Hughes · A.M. Milan · J.A. Gallagher · L.R. Ranganath
Department of Musculoskeletal Biology, Institute of Ageing and
Chronic Disease, William Duncan Building, 6 West Derby Street,
Liverpool L7 8TX, UK

R.M.K. Stewart
Royal Victorian Eye and Ear Hospital, 32 Gisborne St,
East Melbourne, VIC 3002, Australia

E.A. Lock
School of Pharmacy and Biomolecular Sciences, Liverpool John
Moores University, Byrom Street, Liverpool L3 3AF, UK

R.M.K. Stewart
Department of Eye and Vision Science, University of Liverpool,
Liverpool, UK

Introduction

Alkaptonuria (OMIM#203500) is a progressive severe osteo-articular disease with no approved disease modifying therapy to date (Ranganath et al. 2015). Approaches to management are currently symptomatic and palliative and employ ineffective analgesia and surgery, including spinal surgery and joint replacements. The only current hope in terms of disease modification is a drug called nitisinone (Ranganath et al. 2013). Early nitisinone therapy may prevent morbidity; and if started later, it has the potential to slow or arrest disease progression. Nitisinone is not yet licensed for AKU and despite considerable morbidity, AKU is characterised by a relatively normal lifespan. Therefore, safety is an important issue and potential adverse effects are of interest to those involved in the management of metabolic disorders.

AKU is inherited in an autosomal recessive fashion. It is characterised by high circulating homogentisic acid (HGA) due to a genetic defect in the enzyme homogentisate dioxygenase (HGD, EC 1.13.11.5) (Phornphutkul et al. 2002). Ochronosis is the main pathogenetic event in AKU and it results from the conversion of HGA to a polymeric melanin-like pigment that has affinity to connective tissues, especially cartilage (Zannoni et al. 1969). Ochronosis leads to arthritis, valvular heart disease, nephrolithiasis and tendon ruptures (O'Brien et al. 1963).

Nitisinone inhibits p-hydroxyphenyl pyruvate dioxygenase and decreases HGA (Lock et al. 1998). In keeping with the mode of action of nitisinone, circulating tyrosine increases. The tyrosinaemia that occurs during nitisinone treatment resembles hereditary tyrosinaemia type 3. Adverse effects known to be associated with tyrosinaemia include corneal and dermal toxicity (Meissner et al. 2008).

Tyrosinaemia related corneal lesions are reported to be less than 9% in children with hereditary tyrosinaemia type 1 (HT-1) who are treated with nitisinone (Holme and Lindstedt 1998; Gissen et al. 2003). Schauwvlieghe et al. (2013) have reported tyrosine keratopathy in a 16-year-old male who received nitisinone for HT-1. Although corneal symptoms resolved after stopping nitisinone, tyrosine crystals were still detectable in the corneal epithelium using confocal microscopy and slit lamp examination.

Nitisinone has been shown to reduce plasma HGA levels and decrease urinary HGA excretion by greater than 95% in humans (Introne et al. 2011; Ranganath et al. 2016; Milan et al. 2017) and to completely prevent ochronosis in a mouse model of AKU (Preston et al. 2014; Keenan et al. 2015). Since 2012, low dose nitisinone has been used off-label in the NHS England designated National Alkaptonuria Centre (NAC), at the Royal Liverpool University Hospital. Safety monitoring, including annual elective slit lamp examination, is part of the standardised care.

Case Report

A 22-year-old man presented to the NAC in 2012. He had increased circulating and urinary HGA (16.3 μmol/L and 8,416 μmol/L, respectively); as well as two genetic mutations in the HGD loci, consistent with the diagnosis of AKU. Apart from asymptomatic arthropathy of his ankles and feet, he had no other clinical features of AKU. He was also known to have unexplained mild splenomegaly and stable persistent thrombocytopenia. At baseline (V1), a slit

lamp examination of the eye including the cornea was carried out and found to be normal. The visual acuity was 6/4.8 in both eyes. The rest of the physical examination was normal. He was then commenced on nitisinone 2 mg alternate days for 3 months, and then increased to 2 mg daily from month 3 onwards. He was counselled on how to control dietary protein to minimise the rise in serum tyrosine associated with nitisinone treatment. He was advised on an initial 1.0 g/kg protein daily intake to maintain his weight and prevent catabolism. At his visit to the NAC one (V2) and 2 years (V3) after beginning nitisinone 2 mg daily, visual acuity was 6/4.8 in both eyes. Slit lamp examinations were carried out electively and there was no corneal keratopathy. At his third annual visit to the NAC (V4), slit lamp ocular examination revealed typical dendritiform corneal keratopathy in both eyes which was asymptomatic. Visual acuity was 6/5 in the right eye and 6/6 in the left eye. The anterior chamber, iris and lens were all normal. On further questioning, he reported no eye symptoms. Dietary assessment revealed that his dietary protein intake had increased as a result of moving from a predominantly vegetarian diet to relying on take away meals. Nitisinone was stopped and he was given dietary counselling to reduce his protein intake. After 2 weeks, resolution of the dendritic lesion was confirmed on slit lamp examination and nitisinone was restarted at 2 mg daily.

At the annual follow-up visit a year later, namely 4 years after commencing nitisinone (V5), the slit lamp examination showed mild corneal keratopathy in the left eye. Visual acuity was 6/4.8 in each eye; the iris, lens and anterior chamber were all normal. Subjectively, he reported some eye dryness but no eye pain, redness, tearing or visual impairment. The patient also admitted to relapsing in terms of his diet. He was again advised to stop taking nitisinone for 2 months and slit lamp examination was arranged. Table 1 summarises the results of serum tyrosine (sTYR), serum HGA (sHGA), 24 h urinary HGA excretion (uHGA24), weight and dietary protein intake. Figure 1 shows eye photos taken during visits 2–5.

Discussion

To our knowledge, this is the first case describing asymptomatic and in particular painless tyrosine keratopathy in a patient receiving just 2 mg of nitisinone daily. This is expected to influence the monitoring of patients on nitisinone. Incidence of tyrosine keratopathy in AKU patients receiving 2 mg daily dose of nitisinone is estimated at 5% (Introne et al. 2011). In our centre we have over 50 patients on low dose nitisinone and we have reported a case of symptomatic tyrosine keratopathy (Stewart et al. 2014).

Table 1 Summary of the metabolic data for case subject

| | Weight (kg) | BMI (kg/m^2) | Serum measurements (μmol/L) | | 24-h urine measurements | | | Recommended dietary protein intake (g/kg)[a] | Estimated dietary protein intake (g/kg)[b] |
			HGA	Tyrosine	HGA (μmol/ 24 h)	Tyrosine (μmol/ 24 h)	Urine nitrogen[c] (g/kg)		
Baseline (visit 1)	78.2	25.8	16.3	38	17,337	163	–	1.0	1.8
12 months (visit 2)	69.9	22.8	4.6	815	1,487	1,797	0.95	0.8	0.77
24 months (visit 3)	74.3	24.5	10.2	113[d]	1,785	1,357	0.74	0.8	0.78
36 months (visit 4)	74.3	24.5	<3.1	964	1,107	1,912	0.80	0.75	0.98
40 months	–	–	–	745[e]	–	–	–	–	
41 months	–	–	–	578[e]	–	–	–	–	
43 months	–	–	–	518[e]	–	–	–	–	
48 months (visit 5)	79.4	26.2	2.5	841	920	1,354	0.63	0.83	1.1

[a] Represents recommended dietary protein intake
[b] Protein intake was estimated from the patient food diary
[c] Estimated from urinary urea excretion
[d] Nitisinone was not detected in this sample
[e] These were done using blood spot samples

In the literature, there are only two cases describing symptomatic tyrosine keratopathy in AKU patients receiving nitisinone (Table 2). The first case was from a 3-year randomised trial that assessed the safety and efficacy of nitisinone in AKU patients. The affected subject was a 48-year-old male who had symptomatic tyrosine keratopathy after 6 weeks of daily 2 mg nitisinone treatment (Introne et al. 2011). The second case was described by Stewart et al. (2014). The patient was 25-year-old male who experienced typical ocular symptoms of blurred vision, ocular pain, red eyes and epiphora as well as a concomitant urticarial skin rash. He was taking 2 mg nitisinone on alternate days and was not compliant with a low protein diet.

In both published cases of tyrosine corneal keratopathy in AKU, eye symptoms resolved on discontinuation of nitisinone. In the first case, eye symptoms recurred and led to permanent withdrawal of nitisinone; while in the second case, the patient was able to tolerate a once weekly dose of 2 mg. In addition to the two published AKU corneal keratopathy reports, another patient who was commenced on nitisinone 2 mg daily at the NAC, subsequently reported severe symptoms of photophobia, red eye, ocular pain, tearing and visual impairment consistent with tyrosine keratopathy post nitisinone but was then no longer able to be followed up in the NAC (Table 2 summarises the demographics and the clinical features of the four patients).

The lack of pain despite clear corneal involvement in the patient described here is difficult to explain. The cornea is very well innervated and has a rich supply of sensory and autonomic fibres (Muller et al. 2003). Corneal hypoesthesia is well documented in many circumstances including post herpetic infection, corneal surgery, damage to the trigeminal cranial nerve, and systemic conditions such as diabetes (Sacchetti and Lambiase 2014). However, this patient had no such history. The lack of symptoms could be explained by the fact that while the corneal epithelium is well supplied with nerve endings, the underlying stroma is not (Shaheen et al. 2014), and it is tempting to speculate that in this case, if tyrosine deposits were mostly confined to the sub-epithelial stroma, pain would not be a feature. This is supported by descriptions of other stromal lesions of the cornea without the presence of pain (Sacchetti et al. 2016). However, confocal corneal microscopy in a hereditary tyrosinaemia type 2 (HT-2) case has demonstrated the presence of tyrosine crystal in the corneal epithelium even after the resolution of eye symptoms (Kocabeyoglu et al. 2014). Similarly, Schauwvlieghe et al. (2013) described asymptomatic tyrosine corneal deposits in a nitisinone treated HT-1 patient. In both cases the stroma was spared. However, there was no mechanism offered in either report to explain the lack of pain.

Experiments in rats support our speculation to some extent. It is important to remember that the tyrosine concentration in the aqueous humor of the anterior chamber of the eye is much higher than in circulating plasma (Lock et al. 1996). Aqueous humor diffuses into the avascular cornea providing crucial nourishment to the endothelium and stroma. Moreover, due to the unique needs of the eye, concentration of tyrosine is much higher than in plasma. The endothelium on the posterior surface of the cornea is

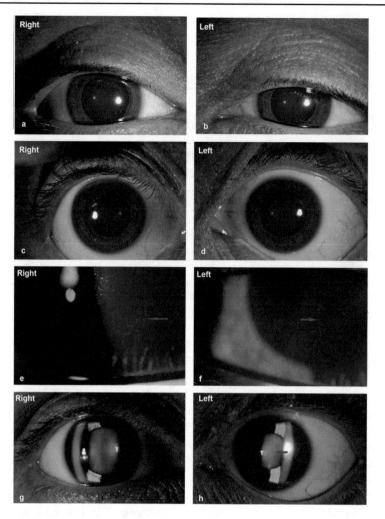

Fig. 1 No evidence of keratopathy in on the first (not shown here), second (**a**, **b**) and third visit (**c**, **d**). On the fourth visit, tyrosine keratopathy lesions are seen in both eyes (red arrows in **e**, **f**).

Fifth visit: Minimal corneal epithelial disturbance with minimal fluorescein uptake in the left eye (red arrow, **h**) and normal right eye (**g**)

leaky compared to the tight epithelium of the anterior corneal surface, allowing the aqueous humor containing the tyrosine to permeate through the cornea stroma. Tyrosine is normally soluble in aqueous humor and precipitates out of solution when its concentrations exceed its solubility in water (Lock et al. 2006). Precipitation of tyrosine in the cornea leads to tyrosine keratopathy. It is likely that the posterior stromal parts of the cornea are exposed to higher tyrosine first and/or affected to a greater extent with a relative sparing the corneal epithelium. This might explain why the richly innervated corneal epithelium is minimally involved, if any, and why symptoms may be lacking.

Serum tyrosine monitoring is important in the context of nitisinone therapy although it may not be very helpful in identifying keratopathy per se. The apparent lack of correlation between serum tyrosine concentrations and eye symptoms has been noted before (Holme and Lindstedt 1998). In a small cohort of nitisinone treated HT-1 children,

there were no ocular symptoms despite non-compliance with low tyrosine diet in four patients and serum tyrosine concentrations were as high as 1,240 and 1,410 μmol/L (Gissen et al. 2003). It can be conjectured that the aqueous humor tyrosine is more meaningful than the circulating tyrosine concentrations.

In this present case, the serum tyrosine concentrations were the highest on the fourth (964 μmol/L) and the fifth visit (841 μmol/L). His dietary protein intake was estimated to be 0.98 g/kg on his fourth visit and 1.1 g/kg on his fifth visit; both consistent with lapses in dietary protein restriction. One could speculate that there may be a correlation between circulating and aqueous humor tyrosine concentrations, in the present case, even though the aqueous humor concentrations were not measured for obvious impractical reasons.

Tyrosine keratopathy can be potentially sight threatening. While there are no reliable predictors of tyrosine keratopathy in AKU patients receiving nitisinone, there are measures that

Table 2 Summary of nitisinone induced tyrosine keratopathy cases in AKU

Case	Age	Gender	Serum tyrosine (μmol/L)	Nitisinone dose	Onset of eye symptoms in relation to starting nitisinone	Outcome	Symptoms
Stewart et al. (2014)	21	Male	941	2 mg alternate days	7 weeks post nitisinone	Restarted nitisinone 2 mg once weekly	Epiphora on alternate evenings while watching television
Introne et al. (2011)	48	Male	600	2 mg daily	6 weeks post nitisinone	Restarting nitisinone attempted twice but eye symptoms recurred	Corneal irritation
Present case	25	Male	964[a] 841[b]	2 mg daily	36 months post nitisinone	Nitisinone 2 mg daily restarted after resolution of keratopathy	No symptoms on visit 4 Dry eyes on visit 5
NAC case (unpublished)	55	Male	1,214	2 mg alternate days	3 months post nitisinone (normal slit lamp examination)	Nitisinone stopped	Experienced right eye discomfort towards the end of the day every other day

[a] Annual visit 4 (V4)
[b] Annual visit 5 (V5)

can be taken to ensure the safe use of nitisinone. Locally, we have a robust protocol for initiating nitisinone and monitoring serum tyrosine concentrations during treatment. Patients are commenced on 2 mg alternate day for 3 months which are then increased to 2 mg daily. Serum tyrosine concentrations are monitored 3 and 6 months after nitisinone initiation and at all annual visits. Patients are counselled regarding low diet tyrosine as well as the potential eye symptoms resulting from hypertyrosinaemia. They are given an alert card and also advised to report eye symptoms promptly and to stop nitisinone. Additionally, ophthalmological assessments are done before starting nitisinone and annually thereafter using slit lamp examination. The present case does not clarify a rationale for frequency of slit lamp examinations required post-nitisinone. It may be necessary to have a higher index of suspicion for potential keratopathy by identifying any atypical or mild ocular symptoms and screening by slit lamp examination. It may also be better to carry out a biannual slit lamp examination. These findings highlight the necessity for further research on managing serum tyrosine concentrations in AKU by dietary or other therapeutic interventions. Further work is also required to elucidate the clinical and prognostic implications of asymptomatic corneal depositions in nitisinone treated patients.

In summary, this is the first case of asymptomatic tyrosine keratopathy in an AKU patient receiving 2 mg daily dose of nitisinone. Elective and symptom-based slit lamp examination may be needed to detect corneal tyrosine keratopathy. Discontinuation of nitisinone, low tyrosine diet and frequent serum tyrosine monitoring remain a key in managing tyrosine keratopathy. The oversight of a meta-

bolic physician and specialised dietary support are paramount.

Take Home Message

Asymptomatic tyrosine keratopathy may occur in AKU patients taking low dose nitisinone. It can be detected using elective and symptom-based slit lamp examination and it should be managed by a metabolic physician and a specialised dietitian.

Compliance with Ethics Guidelines

Conflict of Interest

M. Khedr, S. Judd, M. C. Briggs, A. T. Hughes, A. M. Milan, R. M. K. Stewart, E. A. Lock, J. A. Gallagher and L. R. Ranganath declare that they have no conflict of interest.

Informed Consent

All procedures followed were in accordance with the ethical standards of the responsible committee on human experimentation (institutional and national) and with the Helsinki Declaration of 1975, as revised in 2000 (5). Informed consent was obtained from all patients for being included in the study.

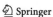

Animal Rights

This article does not contain any studies with human or animal subjects performed by the any of the authors.

Details of the Contributions of Individual Authors

M. Khedr wrote the first draft.

S. Judd carried out dietary assessments.

A. T. Hughes, A. M. Milan, M. C. Briggs, R. M. K. Stewart, E. A. Lock, J. A. Gallagher and L. R. Ranganath: Intellectual input and support, editing the manuscript.

Corresponding Author

M. Khedr.

Guarantor

L. R. Ranganath.

Details of Funding

None.

Details of Ethics Approval

All procedures followed were in accordance with the ethical standards of the responsible committee on human experimentation (institutional and national) and with the Helsinki Declaration of 1975, as revised in 2000. In addition, the institutional review body (Royal Liverpool University Hospital) explicitly approved the National Alkaptonuria Service from which this data was generated.

A Patient Consent Statement

Informed consent was obtained from all patients for being included in the study. This is being published as a clinical practice article and standard research ethics process is not therefore appropriate. The data from this patient have been completely anonymised to ensure he is not recognised from the publication of this manuscript. The data obtained were following standard clinical assessments upon referral to the National Alkaptonuria Service in Liverpool. Patients are informed verbally and through being handwritten materials about the activities of the National AKU Service. They are explicitly informed in the Patient information booklet of the National AKU Service that:

We could publish results from the study but if we do, we will make sure you cannot be identified in any way. All data used for publicity or for other research purposes will ensure total anonymity. Please let us know when you are visiting Ward 9 B (where the National AKU Service is located) that you understand this and have no objection to it.

All the ocular photos were acquired during the standard assessments during the patient visit.

References

Gissen P, Preece M, Willshaw H, McKiernan PJ (2003) Ophthalmic follow-up of patients with tyrosinaemia type I on NTBC. J Inherit Metab Dis 26:13–16

Holme E, Lindstedt S (1998) Tyrosinaemia type I and NTBC (2-(2-nitro-4-trifluoromethylbenzoyl)-1,3-cyclohexanedione). J Inherit Metab Dis 21(5):507–517

Introne WJ, Perry MB, Troendle J et al (2011) A 3-year randomized therapeutic trial of nitisinone in alkaptonuria. Mol Genet Metab 103(4):307–314

Keenan CM, Preston AJ, Sutherland H et al (2015) Nitisinone arrests but does not reverse Ochronosis in Alkaptonuric mice. JIMD Rep 24:45–50

Kocabeyoglu S, Mocan MC, Irkec M (2014) In vivo confocal microscopic features of corneal pseudodendritic lesions in tyrosinemia type II. Cornea 33(10):1106–1108

Lock EA, Gaskin P, Ellis MK et al (1996) Tissue distribution of 2-(2-Nitro-4-trifluoromethylbenzoyl)cyclohexane-1,3-dione (NTBC): effect on enzymes involved in tyrosine catabolism and relevance to ocular toxicity in the rat. Toxicol Appl Pharmacol 141:439–447

Lock EA, Ellis MK, Gaskin P et al (1998) From toxicological problem to therapeutic use: the discovery of the mode of action of 2-(2-nitro-4-trifluoromethylbenzoyl)-1,3-cyclohexanedione (NTBC), its toxicology and development as a drug. J Inherit Metab Dis 21:498–506

Lock EA, Gaskin P, Ellis M, Provan WM, Smith LL (2006) Tyrosinaemia produced by 2-(2-nitro-4-trifluoromethylbenzoyl)-cyclohexane-1,3-dione (NTBC) in experimental animals and its relationship to corneal injury. Toxicol Appl Pharmacol 215:9–16

Meissner T, Betz RC, Pasternak SM et al (2008) Richner-Hanhart syndrome detected by expanded newborn screening. Paediatr Dermatol 25:378–380

Milan AM, Hughes AT, Davison AS et al (2017) The effect of nitisinone on homogentisic acid and tyrosine: a two-year survey of patients attending the National Alkaptonuria Centre, Liverpool. Ann Clin Biochem 54:323–330

Muller LJ, Marfurtb CF, Krusec F, Tervod TM (2003) Corneal nerves: structure, contents and function. Exp Eye Res 76:521–542

O'Brien WM, BNL D, Bunim JJ (1963) Biochemical, pathologic and clinical aspects of alcaptonuria, ochronosis and ochronotic arthropathy. Am J Med 34:813–838

Phornphutkul C, Introne WJ, Perry MB et al (2002) Natural history of alkaptonuria. N Engl J Med 347:2111–2121

Preston AJ, Keenan CM, Sutherland H et al (2014) Ochronotic osteoarthropathy in a mouse model of alkaptonuria, and its inhibition by nitisinone. Ann Rheum Dis 73(1):284–289

Ranganath LR, Jarvis JC, Gallagher JA (2013) Recent advances in management of alkaptonuria (invited review; best practice article). J Clin Pathol 66:367–373

Ranganath LR, Timmis OG, Gallagher JA (2015) Progress in alkaptonuria – are we near to an effective therapy? J Inherit Metab Dis 38:787–789

Ranganath LR, Milan AM, Hughes AT et al (2016) Suitability of nitisinone in alkaptonuria 1 (SONIA 1): an international, multicentre, randomised, open-label, no-treatment controlled, parallelgroup, dose-response study to investigate the effect of once daily nitisinone on 24-h urinary homogentisic acid excretion in patients with alkaptonuria after 4 weeks of treatment. Ann Rheum Dis 75(2):362–367

Sacchetti M, Lambiase A (2014) Diagnosis and management of neurotrophic keratitis. Clin Ophthalmol 8:571–579

Sacchetti M, Macchi I, Tiezzi A, La Cava M, Massaro-Giordano G, Lambiase A (2016) Pathophysiology of corneal dystrophies: from cellular genetic alteration to clinical findings. J Cell Physiol 231:261–269

Schauwvlieghe P-P, Jaeken J, Kestelyn P, Claerhout I (2013) Confocal microscopy of corneal crystals in a patient with hereditary tyrosinemia type I, treated with NTBC. Cornea 32(1):91–94

Shaheen B, Bakir M, Jain S (2014) Corneal nerves in health and disease. Surv Ophthalmol 59(3):263–285

Stewart R, Briggs MC, Jarvis JC et al (2014) Reversible keratopathy due to hypertyrosinaemia following intermittent low-dose nitisinone in alkaptonuria: a case report. JIMD Rep 17:1–6

Zannoni VG, Lomtevas N, Goldfinger S (1969) Oxidation of homogentisic acid to ochronotic pigment in connective tissue. Biochim Biophys Acta 177:94–105

JIMD Reports
DOI 10.1007/8904_2017_61

RESEARCH REPORT

Hyperphenylalaninaemias in Estonia: Genotype–Phenotype Correlation and Comparative Overview of the Patient Cohort Before and After Nation-Wide Neonatal Screening

Hardo Lillevāli · Karit Reinson · Kai Muru ·
Kristi Simenson · Ülle Murumets · Tõnu Möls ·
Katrin Õunap

Received: 06 March 2017 / Revised: 31 August 2017 / Accepted: 04 September 2017 / Published online: 28 September 2017
© Society for the Study of Inborn Errors of Metabolism (SSIEM) 2017

Abstract The present study provides a retrospective overview of the cohort of phenylketonuria (PKU) patients in Estonia. Based on the available data, the patients clearly cluster into two distinct groups: the patients with late diagnosis and start of therapy ($N = 46$), who were born before 1993 when the national newborn screening programme was launched, and the screened babies ($N = 48$) getting their diagnoses at least in a couple of weeks after birth.

Altogether 153 independent phenylalanine hydroxylase (*PAH*) alleles from 92 patients were analysed in the study, wherein 80% of them were carrying the p.Arg408Trp variation, making the relative frequency of this particular variation one of the highest known. Additionally, 15 other different variations in the *PAH* gene were identified, each with very low incidence, providing ground for phenotypic variability and potential response to BH$_4$ therapy. Genealogical analysis revealed some "hotspots" of the origin of the p.Arg408Trp variation, with especially high density in South-East Estonia. According to our data, the incidence of PKU in Estonia is estimated as 1 in 6,700 newborns.

Introduction

Hyperphenylalaninaemia (HPA) is a condition usually caused by the inability of the organism to metabolise phenylalanine (Phe). Most of the HPA cases occur due to variations in the phenylalanine hydroxylase (*PAH*, EC1.14.16.1) gene leading to recessively inherited metabolic disease – phenylketonuria (PKU, OMIM#261600). If untreated, high levels of Phe lead to severe intellectual disability, while early restriction of dietary protein together with the intake of Phe-free substituted protein allows undisturbed mental and physical development (Blau et al. 2010). During the last decades, also tetrahydrobiopterin (BH$_4$) has been introduced to improve the life quality of PKU patients, or substitute dietary treatment in certain cases (Cunningham et al. 2012).

The prevalence of distinct variations in the *PAH* gene varies highly between populations (Zschocke 2003). While in ethnically close Finland PKU is an extremely rare condition (Guldberg et al. 1995), Estonian neighbours Latvia (Pronina et al. 2003) and Lithuania (Kasnauskiene et al. 2003) exhibit similar occurrence and variation structure, also more distant East-European countries like Poland (Bik-Multanowski et al. 2013) and Czech Republic (Reblova et al. 2013); however, oversea neighbours Sweden, Denmark and Norway exhibit much more hetero-

Communicated by: Nenad Blau, PhD

Electronic supplementary material: The online version of this article (https://doi.org/10.1007/8904_2017_61) contains supplementary material, which is available to authorized users.

H. Lillevāli
Institute of Biomedicine and Translational Medicine,
University of Tartu, Tartu, Estonia

H. Lillevāli (✉) · K. Reinson · K. Muru · K. Simenson · Ü. Murumets ·
K. Õunap
Department of Clinical Genetics, United Laboratories,
Tartu University Hospital, Tartu, Estonia
e-mail: hardo.lillevali@kliinikum.ee

K. Reinson · K. Õunap
Department of Clinical Genetics, Institute of Clinical Medicine,
University of Tartu, Tartu, Estonia

T. Möls
Centre for Limnology, Institute of Agricultural and Environmental
Sciences, Estonian University of Life Sciences, Tartu, Estonia

geneous spectra (Eisensmith et al. 1992; Bayat et al. 2016; Ohlsson et al. 2016).

Previously, an overview about the spectrum of PKU allele variations in Estonia has been reported in 1996 in a cohort of 34 PKU patients (Lillevali et al. 1996). Now, we are able to present information about additional 60 PKU patients. The cohort includes new well-documented cases from 1996 to 2016, as well as cases from the period 1974–1996 not included in the previous study.

The aim of the present study is to provide an updated overview of all patients with a HPA diagnosis born and/or living in Estonia since 1974, to update the spectrum of allele variations among persons with HPA, and to gain insight into geographical distribution of the most prevalent variation p.Arg408Trp. We also compare the spectrum of *PAH* gene variations among distinct ethnic groups in Estonia and present corrected data on PKU incidence in Estonia.

Material and Methods

Patient Group

To create the Estonian database about available HPA cases, case histories of the patients born or living in Estonia from 1974 to 2016 were selected and analysed. Data fields with the following aspects were filled: last name as an identifier, year of birth, age and Phe level at diagnosis, method of diagnosis (fluorometrical, tandem mass spectrometry, or Fölling test), highest known Phe concentration value, *PAH* genotype, remarks about medical condition, data about the start and continuation/discontinuation of the treatment, and genealogical data of the patient, including ethnicity of the parents and grandparents of the proband. Additionally, data about general medical/social status of the person were included.

The whole cohort was divided into two subgroups according to the year of birth: 1974–1992 and 1993–2016, i.e. before and after the initiation of national newborn screening programme for PKU in Estonia.

Genealogical Survey

Parents of the PKU patients were requested to fill a questionnaire for genealogical search. It included fields about the names, maiden names, birth dates and birthplaces of the parents and grandparents of the patients, who had at least one grandparent of Estonian ethnic origin.

Prevalence Estimation

Children born during the period from 1993 to 01.09.2016 were taken under observation for estimation of the prevalence of *PAH*-dependent HPA-s in Estonia. Population

data of all live births from 1993 to 2015 was obtained from national agency Statistics Estonia (http://www.stat.ee). The number of screened newborns between 01.01.2016 and 01.09.2016 was added according to the data recorded in the screening laboratory of the Department of Clinical Genetics, United Laboratories of Tartu University Hospital. The data about all Estonian HPA patients were collected at the Department of Clinical Genetics, United Laboratories of Tartu University Hospital.

Mutation Analysis

Mutation analysis of the *PAH* gene of the probands as well as their parents, when available, was performed as described previously (Lillevali et al. 1996) or/and PCR and automated dideoxy sequencing with ABI 3130XL capillary sequencer (Applied Biosystems) of all *PAH* gene NM_000277.1 exons (1–13) and exon–intron boundaries. First, the presence of the prevalent p.Arg408Trp variation was checked, if missing, all *PAH* gene exons were sequenced completely and MLPA analysis was performed using commercially available kit SALSA®MLPA® Probemix P055-*PAH* (MRC-Holland).

Statistical Analysis

Statistical analysis of the genealogical data was performed with SAS software (SAS®9.2 Analytics, SAS Institute Inc.). Data were collected about the birthplaces of the grandparents of PKU patients' parental linage carrying the p.Arg408Trp allele of Estonian ethnicity p.Arg408Trp and determined with the fidelity of county. The analysed dataset consisted of 52 multivariate independent observations corresponding to 52 observed PKU patients. The pool of known localisations contained 162 birthplaces. The number of possible carrier grandparents in each of the 15 counties and the pre-World-War-II Petseri County was normalised to the population number of Estonian ethnicity of each county. Details of the analysis are provided in Supplementary Data 1. Confidence limits to the results were obtained by bootstrap method (Efron 1981).

Results

Description of the Patient Cohort

As a result of the study, a database of 95 records was created. These clustered into two groups according to the period of diagnosis. The first group comprises of 46 patients born between 1974 and 1992, before initiating the national PKU screening programme. These patients can be characterised by delay in diagnosis, mostly at the age between 6 months and 2 years, usually these children were taken under observation after abnormal symptoms had already occurred. This cohort involves also two patients diagnosed at the age of 9 and 11 years. Two late-diagnosed adult PKU patients have escaped intellectual disability. No genetic material and further medical data are available from two emigrated probands. All available genotypes of the patients in the late-diagnosed cohort consisted of homo- or compound heterozygotes for *PAH* alleles with minimal residual *PAH* activity. Nineteen patients continue low-Phe diet in their adulthood. One patient born in 1991 initially diagnosed PKU exhibited no thriving despite low-Phe diet and was subjected to BH$_4$ loading test, unveiling dihydropteridine reductase (DHPR) deficiency.

The second group included 48 children with PKU born since 1993, after the introduction of the screening programme (Ounap et al. 1998). These patients are characterised by early diagnosis, constant observation and medical recordings, and continuous dietary treatment. Their age at diagnosis ranges from 10 to 35 days, with an average value of 24 days. Gradual tendency of earlier diagnosis together with logistical improvement of the screening programme occurred: while the average age of diagnosis in 1993–2000 was 33 days, it decreased to 20 days in 2001–2010, and further to 17 days in 2011–2016. This cohort includes two siblings with mild HPA diagnosed in Belgium, and one foetus prenatally diagnosed and terminated. Clear majority (39) of these patients are prescribed

low-Phe diet and keep it continuously. Four patients receive BH$_4$ supplement to reduce the dietary restrictions, having p.[Arg408Trp];[Leu48Ser], p.[Arg408Trp];[Arg261Gln] and p.[Arg408Trp];[Glu390Gly] genotypes accompanied with milder decrease of *PAH* activity.

PAH Variation Distribution

Genotype data for 92 PKU probands (of 94) was available. Two patients have emigrated, one has died and data about only one of her alleles exist. Mutation analysis of one proband (mild PKU phenotype) has been successful for only one allele. Altogether, we were able to include 182 alleles into the study, 19 of which being related. Accordingly, the known Estonian *PAH* allele pool contains 153 independent alleles. Among these, 123 harboured the p.Arg408Trp variation characteristic to East-European populations, constituting 80.4% of all PKU alleles and thus being one of the highest prevalence reported (Tighe et al. 2003). The full data about *PAH* variations are presented in Table 1.

Ethnical Structure of the Patient Cohort

The ethnical structure of Estonian PKU patients resembles that of the republic. Out of 94 patients, 63 (67%) were Estonians, 24 (26%) Slavic (Russian or Ukrainian) and seven of mixed origin, including Estonian, Latvian,

Table 1 *PAH* variations among PKU patients in Estonia (independent alleles)

Variation in the *PAH* gene	Number of independent alleles	Percentage	Ethnic origin
p.Arg408Trp c.1222C>T	123	80.4	Therein 89 Estonian 31 Slavic 3 Mixed
p Leu48Ser c.143T>C	5	3.3	
p.(?)/IVS12+1G>A c.1315+1G>A	4	2.6	
p.Arg261Gln c.782G>A	3	2	
p.Arg252Trp c.754C>T	2	<1	
p.Glu280Lys c.838G>A	2	<1	
p.Pro281Leu c.842C>T	2	<1	
p.Ile306Val c.916A>G	2	<1	
p.Ile65Thr c.194T>C	1	<1	
p.Arg158Gln c.473G>A	1	<1	
p.Asp222* c.663_664delAG	1	<1	Armenian
p.Ala300Ser c.898G>T	1	<1	
p.Ser349Pro c.1045T>C	1	<1	
p.Glu390Gly c.1169A>G	1	<1	Georgian
p.Gln355_Tyr356insGlyLeuGln/IVS10-11G>A c.1066-11G>A	1	<1	Slavic
p.Ala403Val c.1208C>T	1	<1	Azerbaijan
Unknown (not p.Arg408Trp)	2	1.3	
Total	153	100	

Armenian and Azerbaijan. This structure is highly similar to general Estonian population, which comprises mostly of Estonians (68.8%) and people of East Slavic ethnicities (27.8%), according to Statistics Estonia (http://www.stat.ee) (01.01.2016).

Phenotypic Structure of Estonian HPA Patient Cohort

Vast majority of Estonian PKU patients (87%) exhibit the classical PKU phenotype with high Phe levels if untreated and minimal or zero *PAH* activity. This is in good correlation with the genotypic data, as the variations p.Arg408Trp, p.Arg158Gln, p.Pro281Leu, p.Arg252Trp, p.(?)/IVS12+1G>A (Okano et al. 1991; Danecka et al. 2015) retain negligible residual *PAH* enzymatic activity to the mutated protein. Only nine patients exhibit mild and/or BH$_4$-responsive PKU harbouring p.Arg261Gln, p. Ala403Val, p.Ala300Ser, p.Glu390Gly beside the p. Arg408Trp in the second allele, whereas four patients exhibited good response to BH$_4$ supplementation and are constantly on Kuvan® treatment now. Four patients do

not require treatment. Genotype/phenotype correlation of Estonian HPA patients is presented in Table 2.

Possible Local Origins of P.Arg408Trp Allele Distribution

Statistical analysis of the birthplaces of the grandparents of PKU patients of Estonian ethnicity carrying the p. Arg408Trp variation revealed several counties of Estonia providing higher input of this allele into Estonian *PAH* variation pool. Considering the population density, the local 'hotspot' of p.Arg408Trp locates to three (and one former) counties of Southeastern Estonia, especially to former Petseri County, as well as Võru, Põlva and Valga Counties (3.5, 2.63, 2.04 and 2.01 carrier origins per 10,000 Estonians, respectively), while the number of p.Arg408Trp carrier origins per 10,000 Estonians for the whole country was 0.88. Relatively high input came from Estonian islands, Saaremaa and Hiiumaa, however, with wider confidence limits; a 'hotspot' was also found in Northeastern Ida-Viru County (2.1 carrier origins per 10,000), while Northern, Western mainland and Central Estonia had

Table 2 Allelic combinations and phenotype distribution of Estonian PKU patients

Genotype (mutations in the *PAH* gene)	Number of patients	Frequency (%)	Phenotype
p.[Arg408Trp];[Arg408Trp] c.1222 [C>T];[C>T]	58	62	Classical PKU
p.[Arg408Trp];[Leu48Ser] c.[1222C>T];[143T>C]	4	4.3	3 classical PKU/1 BH$_4$-responsive PKU
p.[Arg408Trp];[(?)/IVS12+1G>A] c.[1222C>T];[1315+1G>A]	3	3.2	Classical PKU
p.[Arg408Trp];[Pro281Leu] c.[1222C>T];[842C>T]	2	2.1	Classical PKU
p.[Arg408Trp];[Arg261Gln] c.[1222C>T];[782G>A]	4	4.3	2 classical PKU/2 BH$_4$-responsive PKU
p.[Arg408Trp];[Glu390Gly] c.[1222C>T];[1169A>G]	1	1.1	BH$_4$-responsive PKU
p.[Arg158Gln];[(?)/IVS12+1G>A] c.[473>A];[1315+1G>A]	1	1.1	Classical PKU
p.[Arg408Trp];[Gln355_Tyr356insGlyLeuGln/IVS10-11G>A] c.[1222C>T];[1066-11G>A]	1	1.1	Classical PKU
p.[Arg408Trp];[Arg252Trp] c.[1222C>T];[754C>T]	4	4.3	Classical PKU
p.[Arg408Trp];[Asp222*] c.[1222C>T];[c.663_664delAG]	2	2.1	Classical PKU
p.[Arg408Trp];[Ser349Pro] c.[1222C>T];[1045T>C]	1	1.1	Classical PKU
p.[Arg408Trp];[Ile306Val] c.[1222C>T];[916A>G]	2	2.1	Mild HPA
p.[Arg408Trp];[Glu280Lys] c.[1222C>T];[838G>A]	2	2.1	Classical PKU
p.[Leu48Ser];[Glu280Lys] c.[143T>C];[838G>A]	1	1.1	Classical PKU
p.[Arg408Trp];[Ile65Thr] c.[1222C>T];[194T>C]	1	1.1	Classical PKU
p.[Arg408Trp];[Ala300Ser] c.[1222C>T];[898G>T]	2	2.1	Mild HPA
p.[Arg408Trp];[Ala403Val] c.[1222C>T];[1208C>T]	1	1.1	Mild PKU
p.[Arg408Trp];[NA] c.[1222C>T];[NA]	1	1.1	Classical PKU
p.[Arg408Trp];[NA] c.[1222C>T];[NA]	1	1.1	Mild PKU
c.[NA];[NA] (no DNA)	2	2.1	Classical PKU
Total	94	100	

relatively few carriers in comparison with their population density (Supplementary Table 1).

The birthplaces of 160 grandparents of PKU patients were marked on a map with red dots and presented in Fig. 1. Each dot shows the origin of p.Arg408Trp with 50% probability.

Prevalence of *PAH* Deficiency

The number of live births in Estonia during 1993 to 01.09.2016 was 321,210. This number was divided with 48, the number of the second sub-cohort of HPA patients, and thus the prevalence of *PAH*-dependent HPA-s in Estonia was estimated as 1 in 6,700. Although some newborns miss from the screening programme due to lack of parental consent, the likelihood of missing a PKU patient from medical observation during last 24 years is negligible; therefore, total national statistics of live births was used. The two probands born in Belgium and one terminated prenatally diagnosed pregnancy were taken into account when determining the prevalence of *PAH*-deficient HPA-s.

Discussion

We present an updated cohort and data about the genotypic and phenotypic distribution of Estonian PKU patients. The relative frequency (80%) of the major p.Arg408Trp variation has remained among the highest across populations, with the most similar prevalence in our mainland neighbour Latvia, followed by Lithuania: 76% and 73.5%, respectively (Kasnauskiene et al. 2003; Pronina et al. 2003), gradually decreasing southward – 62% in Poland, 42% in the Czech Republic (Reblova et al. 2013), 23–27% in Germany (Aulehla-Scholz and Heilbronner 2003), and westward – 14–19% in Sweden (Ohlsson et al. 2016), being also very high (71%) in North-Western direction, the St. Petersburg region (Baranovskaya et al. 1996). The exceptionally high prevalence (84%) of this variation reported two decades ago could be considered a result of insufficient diagnostic capabilities in the past, leaving milder HPA cases out of the reach of paediatricians and clinical geneticists. However, the presence of only six PKU patients exhibiting mild HPA suggests that this could not

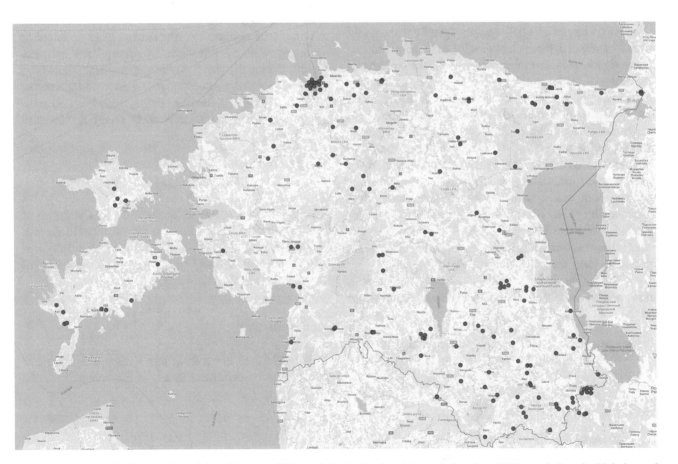

Fig. 1 Geographical distribution of the origins of the p.Arg408Trp variation in the phenylalanine hydroxylase (*PAH*) gene in Estonia. Birthplaces of the grandparents of PKU patients with the p.Arg408Trp variation in the *PAH* gene are shown with red dots. Note that each dot presents 50% probability of the grandparent being a carrier of the variation

have been prevalent. The distribution of this disease-causing allele highly resembles the total genetic structure of various European populations obtained by wide-screen analysis of neutral SNPs (Nelis et al. 2009).

Regional overviews about the diagnostic and management practices have been published lately (Gizewska et al. 2016). In 2012, national guidelines for treatment, diagnostics and management of PKU were approved in Estonia (Uudelepp et al. 2012). These are in good accordance with European guidelines (van Spronsen et al. 2017).

Analysis of the genealogical data and the birthplaces of possible carriers revealed the prevalence of p.Arg408Trp in relatively sparsely populated areas of Southern and Southeastern Estonia. It has been a subject of discussions that heterozygosity for *PAH* deficiency might possess selective advantage, as suggested by the incidence of PKU in distinct populations and with wide diversity in variation spectrum (Krawczak and Zschocke 2003; Zschocke 2003; Saugstad 2006). We speculate for a possible bottleneck effect or genetic drift, as the period of plagues in the seventeenth century and tremendous population loss due to the Great Northern War in the beginning of the eighteenth century may have led to the observed distribution of this particular allele.

Previous research on BH$_4$-responsiveness has shown the need to study each patient individually, as the response may differ significantly due to particular molecular structure of the mutant *PAH* protein. Based on the genotypic structure of Estonian population it is not surprising that our cohort included a small number of BH$_4$-sensitive patients, as is responsible for complete ablation of *PAH* enzymatic activity with no change if excess cofactor provided (Danecka et al. 2015). During the recent 6 years, every HPA newborn has undergone BH$_4$ loading test, while the patients born earlier were not tested. Thus, three older patients with p.[Arg408Trp];[Leu48Ser] genotype are considered as classical PKU and one as BH$_4$ responsive. Now four BH$_4$-responsive patients have been discovered, providing them and their families better life-quality.

In conclusion, Estonia exhibits a notably homogenous pool of disease-causing PKU alleles with high prevalence of the classical severe form of PKU.

Acknowledgements The current study has been supported by grant PUT0355 from the Estonian Science Foundation.

Synopsis

The retrospective overview of Estonian phenylketonuria (PKU) patients revealed that the incidence of PKU in Estonia is 1 in 6,700 newborns with exceptionally high genetic homogeneity, as 80% of all PKU alleles carry the p.Arg408Trp variation typical for Eastern Europe; the genealogical part of the study disclosed certain regions of the country, where said variation was of higher prevalence compared to whole Estonia.

Author Contribution

All the listed authors have contributed to planning, conduct, and writing of the study; the statistical analysis was carried out by Dr. Tõnu Möls.

Guarantor

We declare Prof Katrin Õunap, MD, PhD as guarantor of this study.

Conflict of Interest

Hardo Lilleväli, Karit Reinson, Kai Muru, Kristi Simenson, Ülle Murumets, Tõnu Möls and Katrin Õunap declare that they have no conflict of interest. None of the authors received remunerations or honorariums of any manner or have any relationship that could inappropriately influence results. During the past 5 years the following authors have obtained reimbursement for attending a symposium/conference: K. Õunap (Biomarine, Sanofi, Shire); K. Reinson (Shire), K. Muru (Biomarine, Nutricia, Shire); K. Simenson (Shire).

Compliance with Ethical Standards

This study was approved by Research Ethics Committee of the University of Tartu (approval date 21.09.2015 number 251/T-6). The approval includes obligatory informed consent from all subjects whose personal or genealogical data has been used in the study.

Animal Rights

This article does not contain any studies with human or animal subjects performed by any of the authors.

Funding

The current study has been supported by grant PUT0355 from the Estonian Science Foundation.

Compliance with Ethics Guidelines

This study was approved by Research Ethics Committee of the University of Tartu (approval date 21.09.2015 number 251/T-6).

References

Aulehla-Scholz C, Heilbronner H (2003) Mutational spectrum in German patients with phenylalanine hydroxylase deficiency. Hum Mutat 21:399–400

Baranovskaya S, Shevtsov S, Maksimova S, Kuzmin A, Schwartz E (1996) The mutations and VNTRs in the phenylalanine hydroxylase gene of phenylketonuria in St Petersburg. J Inherit Metab Dis 19:705

Bayat A, Yasmeen S, Lund A, Nielsen JB, Moller LB (2016) Mutational and phenotypical spectrum of phenylalanine hydroxylase deficiency in Denmark. Clin Genet 90:247–251

Bik-Multanowski M, Kaluzny L, Mozrzymas R et al (2013) Molecular genetics of PKU in Poland and potential impact of mutations on BH4 responsiveness. Acta Biochim Pol 60:613–616

Blau N, van Spronsen FJ, Levy HL (2010) Phenylketonuria. Lancet 376:1417–1427

Cunningham A, Bausell H, Brown M et al (2012) Recommendations for the use of sapropterin in phenylketonuria. Mol Genet Metab 106:269–276

Danecka MK, Woidy M, Zschocke J, Feillet F, Muntau AC, Gersting SW (2015) Mapping the functional landscape of frequent phenylalanine hydroxylase (*PAH*) genotypes promotes personalised medicine in phenylketonuria. J Med Genet 52:175–185

Efron B (1981) Nonparametric estimates of standard error: the jackknife, the bootstrap and other methods. Biometrika 68:589–599

Eisensmith RC, Okano Y, Dasovich M et al (1992) Multiple origins for phenylketonuria in Europe. Am J Hum Genet 51:1355–1365

Gizewska M, MacDonald A, Belanger-Quintana A et al (2016) Diagnostic and management practices for phenylketonuria in 19 countries of the South and Eastern European Region: survey results. Eur J Pediatr 175:261–272

Guldberg P, Henriksen KF, Sipila I, Guttler F, de la Chapelle A (1995) Phenylketonuria in a low incidence population: molecular characterisation of mutations in Finland. J Med Genet 32:976–978

Kasnauskiene J, Giannattasio S, Lattanzio P, Cimbalistiene L, Kucinskas V (2003) The molecular basis of phenylketonuria in Lithuania. Hum Mutat 21:398

Krawczak M, Zschocke J (2003) A role for overdominant selection in phenylketonuria? Evidence from molecular data. Hum Mutat 21:394–397

Lillevali H, Ounap K, Metspalu A (1996) Phenylalanine hydroxylase gene mutation R408W is present on 84% of Estonian phenylketonuria chromosomes. Eur J Hum Genet 4:296–300

Nelis M, Esko T, Magi R et al (2009) Genetic structure of Europeans: a view from the north-east. PLoS One 4:e5472

Ohlsson A, Bruhn H, Nordenstrom A, Zetterstrom RH, Wedell A, von Dobeln U (2016) The spectrum of PAH mutations and increase of milder forms of phenylketonuria in Sweden during 1965–2014. JIMD Rep 34:19–26

Okano Y, Eisensmith RC, Güttler F et al (1991) Molecular basis of phenotypic heterogeneity in phenylketonuria. N Engl J Med 324:1232–1238

Ounap K, Lillevali H, Metspalu A, Lipping-Sitska M (1998) Development of the phenylketonuria screening programme in Estonia. J Med Screen 5:22–23

Pronina N, Giannattasio S, Lattanzio P, Lugovska R, Vevere P, Kornejeva A (2003) The molecular basis of phenylketonuria in Latvia. Hum Mutat 21:398–399

Reblova K, Hruba Z, Prochazkova D et al (2013) Hyperphenylalaninemia in the Czech Republic: genotype-phenotype correlations and in silico analysis of novel missense mutations. Clin Chim Acta 419:1–10

Saugstad LF (2006) From genetics to epigenetics. Nutr Health 18:285–300

Tighe O, Dunican D, O'Neill C et al (2003) Genetic diversity within the R408W phenylketonuria mutation lineages in Europe. Hum Mutat 21:387–393

Uudelepp ML, Joost K, Zordania R, Õunap K (2012) Fenüülketonuuria Eesti ravijuhend (Treatment guidelines of phenylketonuria in Estonia; in Estonian). Eesti Arst 91:46–51

van Spronsen FJ, van Wegberg AM, Ahring K et al (2017) Key European guidelines for the diagnosis and management of patients with phenylketonuria. Lancet Diabetes Endocrinol 5 (9):743–756

Zschocke J (2003) Phenylketonuria mutations in Europe. Hum Mutat 21:345–356

JIMD Reports
DOI 10.1007/8904_2017_58

Clinical, Biochemical, and Molecular Features in 37 Saudi Patients with Very Long Chain Acyl CoA Dehydrogenase Deficiency

Abdulrahman Obaid · Marwan Nashabat ·
Majid Alfadhel · Ali Alasmari · Fuad Al Mutairi ·
Abdulrahman Alswaid · Eissa Faqeih ·
Aziza Mushiba · Marwah Albanyan ·
Maryam Alalwan · Deborah Marsden · Wafaa Eyaid

Received: 09 May 2017 / Revised: 28 August 2017 / Accepted: 29 August 2017 / Published online: 05 October 2017
© Society for the Study of Inborn Errors of Metabolism (SSIEM) 2017

Abstract *Background*: Very long chain acyl CoA dehydrogenase (VLCAD) deficiency (OMIM#201475) is an autosomal recessive disorder of fatty acid beta oxidation caused by defect in the *ACADVL*. The aim of this study was to analyze the clinical, biochemical, and molecular features of VLCAD deficiency in Saudi Arabia, including the treatment and outcome.

Methods: We carried out a retrospective chart review analysis of 37 VLCAD deficiency patients from two tertiary centers in Saudi Arabia, over a 14-year period (2002–2016). Twenty-three patients were managed at King Abdul-Aziz Medical City and fourteen patients at King Fahad Medical City.

Results: Severe early onset VLCAD deficiency is the most frequent phenotype in our patients, caused by four different mutations in *ACADVL*; 31 patients (83.7%) had a homozygous nonsense mutation in exon 2 of *ACADVL* c.65C>A;p. Ser22X. Twenty-three patients died before the age of 2 years, despite early detection by newborn screening and implementation of treatment, including supplementation with medium chain triglycerides.

Conclusion: This study reports the clinical, biochemical, molecular findings, treatment, and outcome of patients with VLCAD deficiency over the last 14 years. We identified the most common variant and one new variant in *ACADVL*. Despite early diagnosis and treatment, the outcome of VLCAD deficiency in this Saudi Arabian population remains poor. Preventive measures, such as prenatal diagnosis, could be implemented.

Background

Very long chain acyl CoA dehydrogenase deficiency (VLCAD) is an autosomal recessive disorder of fatty acid beta oxidation, caused by a defect in *ACADVL* gene encoding the VLCAD enzyme, which catalyzes the initial step in the mitochondrial fatty acid beta oxidation pathway (Leslie et al. 1993). This process is essential for energy production during prolonged fasting or periods of increased energy need, such as with intercurrent infection. Dietary long chain fatty acids, or those released from fat stores, are transported into the mitochondria and undergo progressive shortening by a series of chain-length specific enzymes to produce acetyl CoA and beta-hydroxybutyrate (ketones) and reducing equivalents for the mitochondrial respiratory chain, providing an alternate energy source, primarily for the brain and other critical tissues, heart, liver, and skeletal muscle (Vockley and Whiteman 2002; Spiekerkoetter 2010).

Communicated by: Verena Peters

A. Obaid · M. Nashabat · M. Alfadhel · F. Al Mutairi · A. Alswaid ·
M. Albanyan · M. Alalwan · W. Eyaid (✉)
Genetics Division, Department of Pediatrics, King Abdullah International
Medical Research Centre, King Saud bin Abdulaziz University for
Health Science, King Abdulaziz Medical City, Ministry of
National Guard-Health Affairs (NGHA), Riyadh, Saudi Arabia
e-mail: eyaidw@ngha.med.sa

A. Alasmari · E. Faqeih · A. Mushiba
Medical Genetic Section, King Fahad Medical City,
Children's Hospital, Riyadh, Saudi Arabia

D. Marsden
Department of Genetics and Genomics, Boston Children's Hospital,
Boston, MA, USA

VLCAD deficiency was first described in 1985 by Hale et al., and thought to be due to long chain acyl-CoA dehydrogenase deficiency (LCAD) (Hale et al. 1985). In 1993, Aoyama et al. described VLCAD deficiency (Aoyama et al. 1993), and patients previously diagnosed as LCAD were reclassified as VLCAD deficiency. The disease has three heterogeneous clinical phenotypes: severe early onset cardiac and multi-organ failure presenting in the first months of life with dilated or hypertrophic cardiomyopathy, arrhythmia, hepatomegaly, hypoglycemia, and is often lethal; a childhood onset phenotype with hypoketotic hypoglycemia, hepatic dysfunction, and rhabdomyolysis (cardiomyopathy is unlikely); a late onset phenotype, which presents with episodic myopathy and rhabdomyolysis (Andresen et al. 1999).

The diagnosis is established initially by detecting elevations of the C14:1, C14:2, C14, or C12 acylcarnitines (McHugh et al. 2011) on newborn screening or at clinical presentation and may be confirmed by molecular analysis of *ACADVL*. This gene was first cloned in 1995 (Aoyama et al. 1995). Subsequently, hundreds of pathogenic mutations have been discovered. Andresen et al. reviewed potential genotype/phenotype correlation, with a general classification of the pathological mutations: null mutations with no VLCAD enzyme activity, such as truncating variants with severe presentation; missense or single amino acid deletions with residual enzyme activity and milder presentation (Andresen et al. 1999). Diekman et al. reported a strong correlation between LC-FAO flux in fibroblasts and the clinical severity of VLCAD deficiency, suggesting that this assay may have better predictive value compared to enzyme activity or plasma acylcarnitine accumulation (Diekman et al. 2015). There are likely ethnic differences in disease presentation. Most of the reported cases in Andresen et al. were European, with a mild phenotype; however, the cases initially reported by Aoyama et al. from Japan were all of the severe phenotype (Aoyama et al. 1993; Andresen et al. 1999). With the implementation of newborn screening programs, early identification of severe cases has allowed for early management and improved outcomes in some patients. Milder phenotypes may also be detected early, some of whom may remain asymptomatic, but which may reflect the true incidence of the disease (Touma et al. 2001; Spiekerkoetter 2010).

In general, treatment of VLCAD is avoidance of triggers of acute decompensation, such as prolonged fasting and intercurrent infections (catabolic stressors), early intervention for acute symptoms and dietary management, including restriction of long chain fat and supplementation with medium chain triglycerides (MCT) that can diffuse directly into the mitochondria and bypass the enzyme deficiency. Controversially, carnitine supplementation maybe used to help eliminate accumulated organic acid metabolites and prevent a secondary deficiency. Management also requires regular follow up to manage the diet, periodic monitoring of cardiac function and growth parameters (McHugh et al. 2011).

Although Saudi Arabia ranks second globally in the prevalence of genetic diseases (Christianson et al. 2006), this is the first report of clinical outcomes for VLCAD deficiency.

Methods

We carried out a retrospective chart review of 37 cases of VLCAD deficiency identified and followed at two tertiary centers in Saudi Arabia from 2002 to 2016. Twenty-three patients were from King Abdul-Aziz Medical City (KAMC) and 14 patients from King Fahad Medical City (KFMC).

Ethics approval for clinical and laboratory data collection was obtained from the King Abdullah International Medical Research Center (KAIMRC) in Riyadh, Saudi Arabia (RC16/189/R). All patients were detected early by tandem mass spectrometry newborn screening and subsequently treatment with a special metabolic formula containing MCT in addition to carnitine supplementation, with close monitoring and follow up. The diagnosis was confirmed by molecular analysis, including parental carrier testing.

ACADVL was analyzed by PCR and sequencing of coding exon and highly conserved intronic spice sites. The reference sequence of *ACADVL* is NM_000018.3.

Result

Clinical Features

All patients were products of consanguineous marriages. The oldest patient was 6 years old (Table 1). There were 23 female patients and 14 male patients. The female to male ratio was approximately 2:1. The family history of unexplained fetal death was positive in 31 patients (83.7%). Early onset cardiac and multi-organ failure VLCAD deficiency was detected in 27 patients (73%); the childhood hepatic and hypoglycemic form in 8 patients (21.6%); and the periodic myopathic form in 2 patients (5.5%).

Twenty-one patients (56.7%) were found to have a variable degree of hypertrophic cardiomyopathy and one (2%) had dilated cardiomyopathy. Eleven patients (29.7%) had structural heart disease (ventricular and atrial septal defect, pulmonary stenosis, patent ductus arteriosus, or persistent foramen oval). All patients who underwent echocardiogram had normal ejection fraction with a total average at 70.5%.

Table 1 Clinical features

Clinical features		Number of patients	Percentage
Age	0–6 months	14	37.8
	7–18 months	11	29.7
	2–6 years	12	32.4
Sex	Male	14	37.8
	Female	23	62.1
Family history	Positive	31	83.7
	Negative	6	16.2
Phenotype	Severe early onset	27	73
	Hepatic/hypoglycemic	8	21.6
	Myopathic form	2	5.4
Status of health	Deceased	23	62.1
	Alive	14	37.83
Cause of death	Arrhythmia, shock, and multiple organ failure	20	54
	Sudden early onset death	3	8.1
	Rhabdomyolysis and acute kidney injury	1	2.7
Cardiomyopathy	Hypertrophic	21	56.7
	Dilated cardiomyopathy	1	2.7
Structure heart disease	Arterial septal defect	3	8.1
	Ventricular septal defect	3	8.1
	Persistent foramen oval	4	10.8
	Bicuspid aortic valve	1	2.7
	Pulmonary stenosis	1	2.7
Hypotonia	Severe generalized	1	2.7
	Mild to moderate	5	13.5
Hepatomegaly	Predominantly seen	12	32.4
Developmental delay	Severe global developmental delay	1	2.7
	Mild-to-moderate developmental delay	7	18.9
Seizure	Tonic clonic	1	2.7
Others	Nephromegaly	1	2.7

Twelve patients (32.4%) developed hepatomegaly; five patients (13.5%) had hypotonia. Twenty-three (62.1%) died between the ages of 2 days and 3 years. Most deaths were preceded by frequent admissions for metabolic acidosis and rhabdomyolysis. Twenty of them died with multiple organ failure, cardiomyopathy, and arrhythmias. One patient developed acute kidney injury secondary to rhabdomyolysis and three patients (8.1%) died of sudden unexplained death in the first few days of life. Muscular hypotonia was detected in eight patients (21.6%), one of whom also had microcephaly, dysmorphic features, and seizure disorder.

Biochemical Features

All of our cases had high long chain C14 acylcarnitines. Thirty-four (91.9%) had variable elevation of liver enzymes. Five patients (13.5%) had abnormal coagulation profile and twelve patients (32.4%) had mild-to-moderate hypoalbuminemia. Hypoketotic hypoglycemia was detected in 17 patients (46%). Creatine phosphokinase (CPK) was high in 18 cases (48.6%). Recurrent metabolic acidosis was also observed. Most of the biochemical markers increased during metabolic crises.

Molecular Features

Our results showed that the mutational spectrum is narrow with four different mutations in *ACADVL*; 31 patients (83.7%) had a homozygous stop codon nonsense mutation in exon 2 c.65C>A; p.Ser22X (Table 2).

Clinical Outcome

Although all patients received standard treatment regimen mentioned above, including the MCT oil immediately following the diagnosis, the outcome was still poor, with

Table 2 Molecular features

Number of cases	Type of mutation	Exon	Nucleic acid	Protein	Reference	Others
31 patients	Nonsense stop codon	2	c.65C>A (NM_000018.3)	p.Ser22X	Reported by Watanabe et al. (2000)	
2 patients	Nonsense stop codon	3	c.134C>A (NM_000018.3)	P.Ser45X	Reported by Watanabe et al. (2000)	
1 patient	Nonsense substitution	7	c.494T>C (NM_000018.3)	p.Phe165Ser	Unreported	Homozygous variant in exon 4 of ZNF423 c.3250G>A (p.Val1084Ile) (NM_015069.2)
1 patient	Nonsense stop codon		c.1349G>A (NM_000018.3)	p.Arg450His	Fukao et al. (2001)	

recurrent admission for metabolic decompensation, resulting in death in 23 patients (>75% of patients) within first 2 years of life. Two sisters (28 and 18 months) are still alive with good metabolic stability and no cardiomyopathy, and found to have a pathogenic homozygous variant in exon 3 c.134 C>A; p.Ser45x.

A 3-year-old female patient with good metabolic stability was found to have c.1349G>A; p.Arg450His. A new variant in exon 7 c.494T>C; p.Phe165Ser was detected by whole exome sequencing in one 4-year-old female patient who is still alive with severe global developmental delay, generalized hypotonia, and dysmorphic features. This patient had another homozygous probably pathogenic variant in ZNF423 c.3250G>A; p.Val1084Ile. Both variants detected in this patient were also found in heterozygous state in each parent.

Two of the patients who died early had a positive newborn screen and clinical features of VLCAD deficiency and a positive family history but mutation analysis was not obtained.

Discussion

Very long chain Acyl CoA dehydrogenase deficiency is a severe life-threatening metabolic disorder of mitochondrial fatty acid beta-oxidation, which is one of the major metabolic pathways in eukaryotic energy production (Watanabe et al. 2000). The incidence of VLCAD deficiency is between 1:100,000 and 1:120,000 live births (Zytkovicz et al. 2001; Chace et al. 2002) which increased to 1:42,500 after the introduction of tandem MS for expanded newborn screening (Spiekerkoetter et al. 2003). In Saudi Arabia, however, a recent publication reported an incidence of 1:37,000, consistent with other reports of high frequency of metabolic disorders in Saudi Arabia (Alfadhel et al. 2016).

The high consanguinity rate among Saudi population (Al-Gazali et al. 2006) could explain the high incidence of the disease.

It is apparent from our study and previous reports that VLCAD deficiency is a clinically heterogeneous disease that can be divided into three major phenotypes as previously described (Ogilvie et al. 1994; Andresen et al. 1999). Most of our patients presented with a severe early onset cardiac and multi-organ failure phenotype in the first few months of life, mainly in the neonatal period. Despite dietary modification and frequent monitoring, the mortality rate was 62%. The overall mortality rate of VLCAD deficiency was reported previously to reach up to 75% (Andresen et al. 1999) in clinically diagnosed patients, prenewborn screening. The poor outcome in our study is likely related to the severe null mutations in a consanguineous population. The majority of the severe cases in our cohort were cardiomyopathic; however, there was no correlation between the degree of cardiomyopathy and the ejection fraction, and death. It is possible that arrhythmias played important role in sudden death of our patients. Arrhythmias have been previously reported in VLCAD deficiency patients. These include QT prolongation, polymorphic ventricular tachycardia, and ventricular fibrillation, sometimes without cardiomyopathy (Bonnet et al. 1999; Gelinas et al. 2011; Yamamoto et al. 2013).

A stop codon variant c.65C>A; p.Ser22X was found in 84% of our patients. This null mutation was initially described by Watanabe et al. and encodes a truncated protein leading to a complete deficiency of the VLCAD enzyme (Andresen et al. 1999; Watanabe et al. 2000).

The null mutation, reported by Touma et al., with a relatively milder cardiomyopathy phenotype, was also found in our population, but despite early diagnosis and treatment, the outcome was poor.

Interestingly, the c.134 C>A (p.Ser45X), nonsense mutation was detected in two patients with good metabolic control and no cardiomyopathy. As for the c.65C>A nonsense variant, the encoding VLCAD protein should be completely deficient. The relatively good metabolic health in the patient with the c.134C>A mutation is therefore probably explained by other genetic or environmental factors. The other previously reported mutation, c.1349G>A p.Arg450His, was detected in a 3-year-old patient. It was previously reported in a 14-year-old Japanese girl (Fukao et al. 2001) as a compound heterozygote, with residual activity and a milder phenotype, similar to our patient.

In this study we also report a new variant, which was identified by WES, the variant, c.494T>C (p.Phe165Ser) in exon 7 of *ACADVL*, affect a highly conserved amino acid, and introduce a large physiochemical deference. Indeed, in silico analysis predicted that this variant was pathogenic. Another variant in exon 4 of the *ZNF423* c.3250G>A; p.Val1084Ile (associated with Joubert syndrome type 19 [OMIM # 614884]) was detected and could explain the unexpected phenotypes in this particular patient.

We did not detect any patient in this study with the variant c.848T>C; p.V283A, reported in the literature as the most frequent mutation in VLCAD deficient patients (Miller et al. 2015; Evans et al. 2016). This variant is often associated with residual enzyme activity and mild hepatopathic (hypoglycemia may occur) or episodic myopathic adult form of VLCAD deficiency that responds well to standard treatment (Andresen et al. 1999; Touma et al. 2001; Miller et al. 2015). The new variant detected in this study broadens the genetic spectrum of VLCAD deficiency; however, the detection of another homozygous variant in *ZNF423* may indicate presence of another genetic disease in this patient which is not uncommon in our society. Al-Owain et al. discussed the concept of "Double hit" and reported many examples of patients with two or more concurrent genetic diseases as in our patient population, which was attributed to the high rate of consanguinity in Saudi society (Al-Owain et al. 2012).

The presence of a common null mutation in our patients and the poor outcome despite early diagnosis and treatment suggests that preventive measures may be an option. In our centers, in addition to thorough genetic counseling for affected families, we offer prenatal diagnosis for future pregnancies. With education and the philosophy that the "current patient is the last patient in the family," most of the families accept the offered preventive measures.

Conclusion

In our retrospective study of 37 VLCAD deficiency patients over a 14-year period, the clinical outcomes and genotypes in our patients are different to that reported in the Caucasian population, with majority of cases having a severe early onset cardiac and multi-organ failure phenotype. Homozygosity for the c.65C>A nonsense mutation is the common with 83.7% of cases. Despite the early detection by newborn screening and early implementation of standard treatment, the outcome is fatal in most patients in the first 2 years of life. The prevention of this disease in our population may require pre-implantation genetic diagnosis, prenatal genetic testing, and carrier testing of high risk family members in addition to premarital genetic carrier testing for the known family mutation.

Acknowledgments The authors would like to thank the patients and their families. The authors would also like to extend their acknowledgment to Ms. Rasha Al-kindi for her support in data collection.

Learning Point

Truncating null mutations was the most common genotype in our VLCAD deficiency patients, with poor outcome despite early diagnosis and proper management. Prenatal diagnosis be a preferable strategy for managing this disorder in our population.

Details of the Contributions of Individual Authors

AO: performed the majority of work associated with preparing, writing, and submitting the manuscript and contributed to the clinical diagnosis and management of the patient. MN: performed work associated with preparing, writing, and intellectual discussion. MF, AAS, and FM: contributed to the diagnosis and management of the patient at KAMC and edited the manuscript. AAA, EF, and AM: contributed to the clinical diagnosis and management of the patient at KFMC and edited the manuscript. DM: Study design, manuscript writing, and final revision. MAB and MAA: Data collection and manuscript revision. WE: contributed to the clinical diagnosis and management of the patient and performed the work related to study design, conceptual discussion, and manuscript writing and revision. All authors read and approved the final manuscript.

Guarantor Author

Wafaa Eyaid.

Compliance with Ethics Guidelines

Conflict of Interest

Abdulrahman Obaid, Marwan Nashabat, Majid Alfadhel, Ali Alasmari, Fuad Al Mutairi, Abdulrahman Alswaid, Eissa Faqeih, Aziza Mushiba, Deborah Marsden, Marwah Albanyan, Maryam Alalwan, and Wafaa Eyaid declare that they have no conflict of interest.

Informed Consent

All procedures followed were in accordance with the ethical standards of the responsible committee on human experimentation (institutional and national) and with the Helsinki Declaration of 1975, as revised in 2000 (5). Informed consent was obtained from all parents and available upon request.

Details of Ethics Approval

This study was approved by King Abdullah International Medical Research Center IRB (RC16/189/R).

Details of Funding

This study received no specific funding from any financial support agency either public or commercial and not-for-profit sectors.

References

Alfadhel M, Benmeakel M, Hossain MA et al (2016) Thirteen year retrospective review of the spectrum of inborn errors of metabolism presenting in a tertiary center in Saudi Arabia. Orphanet J Rare Dis 11:126

Al-Gazali L, Hamamy H, Al-Arrayad S (2006) Genetic disorders in the Arab world. BMJ 333:831–834

Al-Owain M, Al-Zaidan H, Al-Hassnan Z (2012) Map of autosomal recessive genetic disorders in Saudi Arabia: concepts and future directions. Am J Med Genet A 158A:2629–2640

Andresen BS, Olpin S, Poorthuis BJ et al (1999) Clear correlation of genotype with disease phenotype in very-long-chain acyl-CoA dehydrogenase deficiency. Am J Hum Genet 64:479–494

Aoyama T, Uchida Y, Kelley RI et al (1993) A novel disease with deficiency of mitochondrial very-long-chain acyl-CoA dehydrogenase. Biochem Biophys Res Commun 191:1369–1372

Aoyama T, Souri M, Ueno I et al (1995) Cloning of human very-long-chain acyl-coenzyme a dehydrogenase and molecular characterization of its deficiency in two patients. Am J Hum Genet 57:273–283

Bonnet D, Martin D, De Pascale L et al (1999) Arrhythmias and conduction defects as presenting symptoms of fatty acid oxidation disorders in children. Circulation 100:2248–2253

Chace DH, Kalas TA, Naylor EW (2002) The application of tandem mass spectrometry to neonatal screening for inherited disorders of intermediary metabolism. Annu Rev Genomics Hum Genet 3:17–45

Christianson A, Howson CP, Modell B (2006) March of Dimes global report on birth defects: the hidden toll of dying and disabled children. In: March of Dimes global report on birth defects: the hidden toll of dying and disabled children. March of Dimes Birth Defects Foundation, White Plains, p 76

Diekman EF, Ferdinandusse S, van der Pol L et al (2015) Fatty acid oxidation flux predicts the clinical severity of VLCAD deficiency. Genet Med 17:989–994

Evans M, Andresen BS, Nation J, Boneh A (2016) VLCAD deficiency: follow-up and outcome of patients diagnosed through newborn screening in Victoria. Mol Genet Metab 118:282–287

Fukao T, Watanabe H, Orii K et al (2001) Myopathic form of very-long chain acyl-CoA dehydrogenase deficiency: evidence for temperature-sensitive mild mutations in both mutant alleles in a Japanese girl. Pediatr Res 49:227–231

Gelinas R, Thompson-Legault J, Bouchard B et al (2011) Prolonged QT interval and lipid alterations beyond beta-oxidation in very long-chain acyl CoA dehydrogenase null mouse hearts. Am J Physiol Heart Circ Physiol 301:H813–H823

Hale DE, Batshaw ML, Coates PM et al (1985) Long-chain acyl coenzyme a dehydrogenase deficiency: an inherited cause of nonketotic hypoglycemia. Pediatr Res 19:666–671

Leslie ND, Valencia CA, Strauss AW, Connor JA, Zhang K (1993) Very long-chain acyl-coenzyme A dehydrogenase deficiency. In: Pagon RA, Adam MP, Ardinger HH et al (eds) GeneReviews®. University of Washington, Seattle, Seattle

McHugh D, Cameron CA, Abdenur JE et al (2011) Clinical validation of cutoff target ranges in newborn screening of metabolic disorders by tandem mass spectrometry: a worldwide collaborative project. Genet Med 13:230–254

Miller MJ, Burrage LC, Gibson JB et al (2015) Recurrent *ACADVL* molecular findings in individuals with a positive newborn screen for very long chain acyl CoA dehydrogenase (VLCAD) deficiency in the United States. Mol Genet Metab 116:139–145

Ogilvie I, Pourfarzam M, Jackson S, Stockdale C, Bartlett K, Turnbull DM (1994) Very long-chain acyl coenzyme a dehydrogenase deficiency presenting with exercise-induced myoglobinuria. Neurology 44:467–473

Spiekerkoetter U (2010) Mitochondrial fatty acid oxidation disorders: clinical presentation of long-chain fatty acid oxidation defects before and after newborn screening. J Inherit Metab Dis 33:527–532

Spiekerkoetter U, Tenenbaum T, Heusch A, Wendel U (2003) Cardiomyopathy and pericardial effusion in infancy point to a fatty acid b-oxidation defect after exclusion of an underlying infection. Pediatr Cardiol 24:295–297

Touma EH, Rashed MS, Vianey-Saban C et al (2001) A severe genotype with favourable outcome in very long chain acyl CoA dehydrogenase deficiency. Arch Dis Child 84:58–60

Vockley J, Whiteman DA (2002) Defects of mitochondrial beta-oxidation: a growing group of disorders. Neuromuscul Disord 12:235–246

Watanabe H, Orii KE, Fukao T et al (2000) Molecular basis of very long chain acyl CoA dehydrogenase deficiency in three Israeli patients: identification of a complex mutant allele with P65L and K247Q mutations, the former being an exonic mutation causing exon 3 skipping. Hum Mutat 15:430–438

Yamamoto A, Nakamura K, Matsumoto S et al (2013) VLCAD deficiency in a patient who recovered from ventricular fibrillation, but died suddenly of a respiratory syncytial virus infection. Pediatr Int 55:775–778

Zytkovicz TH, Fitzgerald EF, Marsden D et al (2001) Tandem mass spectrometric analysis for amino, organic, and fatty acid disorders in newborn dried blood spots: a two-year summary from the New England Newborn Screening Program. Clin Chem 47: 1945–1955

JIMD Reports
DOI 10.1007/8904_2017_57

RESEARCH REPORT

Novel Missense LCAT Gene Mutation Associated with an Atypical Phenotype of Familial LCAT Deficiency in Two Portuguese Brothers

I. Castro-Ferreira · Rute Carmo · Sérgio Estrela Silva ·
Otília Corrêa · Susana Fernandes · Susana Sampaio ·
Rodrigues-Pereira Pedro · Augusta Praça ·
João Paulo Oliveira

Received: 01 August 2017 / Revised: 27 August 2017 / Accepted: 29 August 2017 / Published online: 06 October 2017
© Society for the Study of Inborn Errors of Metabolism (SSIEM) 2017

Abstract Familial lecithin-cholesterol acyltransferase deficiency (FLD) is a rare recessive disorder of cholesterol metabolism, caused by loss-of-function mutations in the human LCAT gene, leading to alterations in the lipid/lipoprotein profile, with extremely low HDL levels.

The classical FLD phenotype is characterized by diffuse corneal opacification, haemolytic anaemia and proteinuric chronic kidney disease (CKD); an incomplete form, only affecting the corneas, has been reported in a few families worldwide.

We describe an intermediate phenotype of LCAT deficiency, with CKD preceding the development of corneal clouding, in two Portuguese brothers apparently homozygous for a novel missense LCAT gene mutation. The atypical phenotype, the diagnosis of membranous nephropathy in the proband's native kidney biopsy, the late-onset and delayed recognition of the corneal opacification, the co-segregation with Gilbert syndrome and the late recurrence of the primary disease in kidney allograft all contributed to obscure the diagnosis of an LCAT deficiency syndrome for many years.

Communicated by: Robert Steiner

I. Castro-Ferreira · R. Carmo · S. Sampaio · A. Praça
Service of Nephrology, Centro Hospitalar São João, Alameda Prof.
Hernâni Monteiro, 4200-319 Oporto, Portugal
e-mail: rute.carvalho.carmo@gmail.com; susana.sampaio@sapo.pt;
augustapraca@gmail.com

I. Castro-Ferreira (✉) · S. Fernandes · S. Sampaio · J.P. Oliveira
I3S – Instituto de Investigação e Inovação em Saúde, Universidade do
Porto, Rua Alfredo Allen 208, 4200-135 Oporto, Portugal
e-mail: inescastroferreira@sapo.pt; sf@med.up.pt; susana.
sampaio@sapo.pt; jpo@med.up.pt

S.E. Silva
Service of Ophthalmology, Centro Hospitalar São João, Alameda Prof.
Hernâni Monteiro, 4200-319 Oporto, Portugal
e-mail: sestrelasilva@gmail.com

S.E. Silva
Department of Organs of the Senses, Faculdade de Medicina da
Universidade do Porto, Alameda Prof. Hernâni Monteiro, 4200-319
Oporto, Portugal
e-mail: sestrelasilva@gmail.com

O. Corrêa
Labco Clinical Laboratory Dr. João Ribeiro, Rua Augusto Simões,
1430 - 1°, salas 1-3, 4470-147 Maia, Portugal
e-mail: Otilia.correa@labco.eu

S. Fernandes
Unit of Genetics, Department of Pathology, Faculdade de Medicina da
Universidade do Porto, Alameda Prof. Hernâni Monteiro, 4200-319
Oporto, Portugal
e-mail: sf@med.up.pt

R.-P. Pedro
Service of Pathology, Centro Hospitalar São João, Alameda Prof.
Hernâni Monteiro, 4200-319 Oporto, Portugal
e-mail: pe_r_pereira@hotmail.com

R.-P. Pedro
Department of Pathology, Faculdade de Medicina da Universidade do
Porto, Alameda Prof. Hernâni Monteiro, 4200-319 Oporto, Portugal
e-mail: pe_r_pereira@hotmail.com

A. Praça · J.P. Oliveira
NephroCare Haemodialysis Clinic, Rua João Mendes Cardoso, 24-C,
4520-233 Santa Maria da Feira, Portugal
e-mail: augustapraca@gmail.com; jpo@med.up.pt

J.P. Oliveira
Service of Medical Genetics and Reference Centre for Inherited
Metabolic Diseases, Centro Hospitalar São João, Alameda Prof.
Hernâni Monteiro, 4200-319 Oporto, Portugal
e-mail: jpo@med.up.pt

A major teaching point is that on standard light microscopy examination the kidney biopsies of patients with LCAT deficiency with residual enzyme activity may not show significant vacuolization and may be misdiagnosed as membranous nephropathy. The cases of these two patients also illustrate the importance of performing detailed physical examination in young adults presenting with proteinuric CKD, as the most important clue to the diagnosis of FLD is in the eyes.

Introduction

Lecithin-cholesterol acyltransferase (LCAT) is a plasma enzyme essential for the esterification of free cholesterol (Kuivenhoven et al. 1997; Kunnen and Van Eck 2012). LCAT reacts with preβ1-HDL containing apolipoprotein A-I (apoA1), where it esterifies free cholesterol via α-LCAT activity; a lesser amount of the enzyme circulates bound to apolipoprotein B in low-density lipoproteins (LDL) and very low-density lipoproteins (VLDL), where it esterifies cholesterol via β-LCAT activity. LCAT also plays an important role in the reverse cholesterol transport pathway.

The LCAT gene is located on chromosome 16q22.1 and comprises 6 exons (OMIM*606967; http://omim.org/entry/606967). LCAT mutations cause two very rare autosomal recessive disorders: Familial LCAT Deficiency (FLD or Norum disease; OMIM#245900; http://omim.org/entry/245900), and Fish-Eye Disease (FED; OMIM#136120; http://omim.org/entry/136120). The Human Gene Mutation Database (HGMD®) currently compiles 102 functionally relevant LCAT variants, including 77 missense/nonsense point mutations (http://www.hgmd.cf.ac.uk; last accessed on August 1, 2017).

FLD is characterized by diffuse corneal opacification, haemolytic anaemia, proteinuria and chronic kidney disease (CKD) (Kuivenhoven et al. 1997; Santamarina-Fojo et al. 2001). Corneal opacities arise in childhood and worsen with age, eventually causing severe sight impairment, sometimes requiring corneal transplantation. Proteinuria develops early, but azotaemia is usually detected only after the second decade of life, progressing to nephrotic proteinuria and end-stage renal disease (ESRD) by the fourth decade. The FLD-associated nephropathy also recurs in kidney allografts (Panescu et al. 1997; Strom et al. 2011; Hui Liew et al. 2016). In FLD, α- and β-LCAT activities are suppressed, leading to high levels of unesterified cholesterol and extremely low levels of high-density lipoproteins (HDL). LDL levels are also low, with normal or increased triglyceride levels. Cholesterol-laden foam-cells and membrane-bound vesicles accumulate in the corneas, kidneys, liver, spleen, bone marrow and arteries. However, hepato-megaly, splenomegaly and lymphadenopathy have been rarely reported and the risk for coronary heart disease is only modestly increased (Santamarina-Fojo et al. 2001; Calabresi et al. 2009).

FED presents a milder phenotype, with predominant involvement of the cornea, without anaemia or CKD. Plasma triglyceride levels are normal to increased and HDL is decreased, due to a partial deficiency of α-LCAT activity (Kuivenhoven et al. 1997). Since β-LCAT activity is preserved, the cholesterol esterification rate and the percentage of cholesteryl esters in plasma are normal. Intermediate, atypical phenotypes have also been described (Kuivenhoven et al. 1997).

The lipid/lipoprotein profile is indistinguishable between subjects classified as FLD or FED, and significantly low levels of HDL and apoA1 are a hallmark of both disorders (Calabresi et al. 2005).

Although the pathogenesis of glomerulosclerosis and progressive CKD in FLD is not well understood, renal accumulation of lipoprotein-X (Lp-X) is probably a major factor contributing to the development of glomerular basement membrane (GBM) and endothelial damage, podocyte effacement, expansion of the mesangial matrix and renal tubule vacuolation. Lp-X is a multilamellar vesicle enriched in free cholesterol, and relatively devoid of cholesterol esters, triglycerides and apolipoproteins; notably, due to the residual activity of LCAT, it does not accumulate in FED. In cell culture studies, Lp-X was found to be cytotoxic and pro-inflammatory (Lynn et al. 2001), and its chronic administration to LCAT$^{-/-}$ knock-out (KO) mice results in accumulation of Lp-X in the kidney, recapitulating most of the renal pathological hallmarks of FLD and the onset of proteinuria (Ossoli et al. 2016).

Genotype–phenotype correlations have been difficult to establish, since affected relatives may have different clinical and biochemical manifestations (Calabresi et al. 2005). Diagnosis of LCAT deficiency may be difficult to recognize, particularly in patients with atypical phenotypes.

Herein, we report on two brothers presenting with an intermediate phenotype of LCAT deficiency-associated with a novel LCAT gene mutation, in which the interpretation of the biochemical laboratory data was confounded by co-segregation of LCAT deficiency with Gilbert syndrome.

Case Reports and Family Data

Patient 1: The Proband

Hypertension and proteinuric CKD were incidentally recognized in this patient at age 26 years, warranting referral to a nephrology clinic for further assessment. The baseline laboratory workup showed moderate normochromic/normocytic anaemia, mild thrombocytopenia, azotaemia (plasma creatinine (pCr): 1.6 mg/dL), erythrocyturia and nephrotic proteinuria (6.88 g/24 h), with normal results of protocol immunological and serological testing. Membranous nephropathy was suggested by kidney biopsy, but its evaluation had been restricted to routine light microscopy (LM). Although the proband had a mildly intellectually disabled older brother who also suffered from advanced CKD with massive proteinuria (Fig. 1), investigation for an underlying hereditary disorder was not pursued.

Regular haemodialysis treatment was started at age 33 and, 5 years afterwards, following notice of progressive clouding of both corneas causing visual impairment and referral for ophthalmological examination (Fig. 2a), the diagnosis of LCAT deficiency (Fig. 2b) was eventually established. The patient's lipid and lipoprotein profile was characterized by low levels of HDL and apoA1, with a normal ratio of free to esterified cholesterol (Fig. 2c). In addition, persistent unconjugated hyperbilirubinemia with normal plasma levels of other liver function tests, lactate dehydrogenase and haptoglobin, an unremarkable peripheral blood smear and negative Coombs test, was suggestive of Gilbert syndrome. The liver and spleen were not palpable by physical examination and presented normal sizes on the ultrasound scan.

Sequence analysis of all the exons and corresponding exon–intron boundaries of the LCAT gene revealed a c.803G>T transition in exon 6, leading to a novel non-conservative substitution of arginine by leucine on amino acid

position 268 of the LCAT protein – i.e., p.(Arg268Leu) – apparently in homozygosity. In addition, genetic analysis of the 5' promoter region of the uridine 5'-diphosphoglucuronosyltransferase gene (UGT1A1) showed (apparent) homozygosity for the longer A(TA)7TAA variant of the TATAA element, confirming the diagnosis of Gilbert syndrome.

At age 40, the patient received a deceased-donor kidney allograft. The post-transplant period was uneventful for several years, with stable graft function (pCr: 1 mg/dL) and without anaemia, proteinuria or microscopic haematuria, under maintenance triple-drug immunosuppression with prednisolone, tacrolimus and mycophenolate mofetil. The abnormal lipid profile and unconjugated hyperbilirubinemia did not resolve after kidney transplantation and a bone marrow aspirate, obtained for the investigation of unremitting thrombocytopenia, did not show any relevant abnormalities, including foam cells or sea-blue histiocytes. Noncontact in vivo confocal laser scanning microscopy for high resolution imaging of all corneal layers revealed diffuse hyperreflectivity of the corneal stroma, due to coalescence of multiple hyperreflective spots (Fig. 3a, b).

Recurrence of haematuria and proteinuria (1.7 g/24 h) supervened during the fifth year post-transplant, prompting an allograft biopsy, whilst the pCr concentration remained within normal range. The transplant kidney biopsy showed the typical histopathological and ultrastructural features of FLD-associated nephropathy (Fig. 3c, d). Treatment with a renin-angiotensin-aldosterone system (RAAS) inhibitor led to partial resolution of proteinuria, but the haematuria

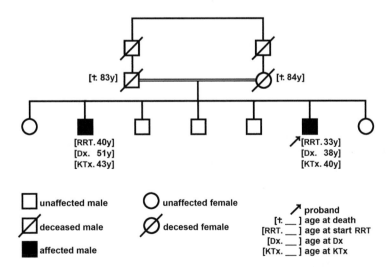

Fig. 1 Family pedigree. The proband is the youngest male of 7 sibs, whose parents were first-cousins. Five of the sibs reported no health problems. Only the mother and the older sister accepted to be screened for manifestations of LCAT deficiency and CKD: none of them showed corneal clouding and their laboratory workups were entirely normal, including the peripheral blood counts as well as the serum lipid profile and the apolipoprotein A–I level. None of the patients' relatives accepted genetic screening. Both parents eventually died aged over 80. Ages are reported in full years. *y* years, *RRT* renal replacement therapy, *KTx* kidney transplantation, *Dx* LCAT deficiency diagnosis, † death

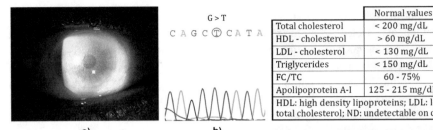

	Normal values	Proband	Brother	Mother	Sister
Total cholesterol	< 200 mg/dL	92	98	227	185
HDL - cholesterol	> 60 mg/dL	12	17	43	33
LDL - cholesterol	< 130 mg/dL	ND	ND	(---)	(---)
Triglycerides	< 150 mg/dL	89	74	114	87
FC/TC	60 - 75%	69	(---)	(---)	(---)
Apolipoprotein A-I	125 - 215 mg/dL	45	(---)	139	194

HDL: high density lipoproteins; LDL: low density lipoproteins; FC/TC: free cholesterol / total cholesterol; ND: undetectable on direct measurement; (---): not measured

a)   b)   c)

Fig. 2 (**a**) Dystrophic corneal opacity; (**b**) DNA electropherogram of the relevant sequence showing apparent homozygosity for a c.803G>T transition in exon 6, leading to a novel non-conservative substitution of arginine by leucine on amino acid position 268 of the LCAT protein – i.e., p.(Arg268Leu); (**c**) Summary of the lipid profiles of the patients and some of their relatives

persisted and mild azotaemia (pCr: 1.4 mg/dL) was detected for the first time.

Case 2: The Proband's Older Brother

When the diagnosis of LCAT deficiency was established in the proband, his older brother, then aged 51, was on the eighth year post-kidney transplantation, undergoing maintenance triple-drug immunosuppression with prednisolone, cyclosporine and mycophenolate mofetil.

The patient's previous renal history was relevant for high blood pressure known since his mid-thirties followed, at age 38, by diagnosis of CKD (pCr: 2.5 mg/dL) with nephrotic syndrome. Kidney biopsy was not performed due to the advanced renal disease. Additional relevant baseline laboratory findings included moderate normochromic/normocytic anaemia and mild thrombocytopenia. Bilateral, slight corneal clouding had already been noticed, but did not prompt appropriate ophthalmological evaluation. Regular haemodialysis treatment was initiated 2 years after, and at the age of 43, the patient received a deceased-donor kidney allograft.

The diagnosis of LCAT deficiency in his younger brother led to a targeted review of the patient's medical records, which showed a serum lipid profile similar to that of the proband (Fig. 1c), as well as persistent mild thrombocytopenia and unconjugated hyperbilirubinemia, without other blood cytopaenias, evidence of chronic liver disease or of chronic haemolysis. Sequencing analyses of the LCAT exon 6 and of the UGT1A1 5' promoter region revealed the same genetic makeup as in his brother.

During the 12th post-transplantation year, the new development of microscopic haematuria and proteinuria (3.69 g/24 h), without allograft dysfunction (pCr: 0.97 mg/dL), prompted a diagnostic allograft biopsy, which documented the recurrence of FLD-associated nephropathy (Fig. 3e, f), even before than in his younger brother.

The patient's subsequent clinical course was marked by severe, badly controlled hypertension; persistent proteinuria, despite upward dose titration of the RAAS inhibitor; many hospitalizations due to infectious complications; and rapid decline of the allograft function, reaching a pCr of 1.62 mg/dL at 14th year post-transplantation.

Discussion

We describe an intermediate clinical phenotype of FLD in two brothers who are (apparently) homozygous for a novel LCAT missense variant, concordantly predicted to be deleterious on bioinformatic analyses using the online software tools MutationTaster (http://www.mutationtaster. org), Polyphen-2 (http://genetics.bwh.harvard.edu/pph2/) and SIFT (http://sift.jcvi.org/). Although parental heterozygosity for the p.(Arg268Leu) LCAT variant could not be directly demonstrated, their consanguineous condition and the rarity of LCAT deficiency in the general population are strong indirect evidence in favour of homozygosity. A further argument against the alternative explanation of compound heterozygosity with a large deletion involving the exon 6 of LCAT, not identifiable on routine DNA sequencing, is that no such type of mutation has so far been reported to the HGMD®. Three other missense mutations, all of them described in patients presenting with FLD, have been reported to affect the same LCAT codon – p.(Arg268Gly) (Skretting et al. 1992), p.(Arg268His) (Calabresi et al. 2005) and p.(Arg268Cys) (Charlton-Menys et al. 2007).

Our patients presented with clinical features of renal involvement that are typical of FLD. The significant age difference at the beginning of haemodialysis illustrates the phenotypic variation of LCAT deficiency within affected families (Skretting et al. 1992). However, the late presentation of corneal opacification and the absence of haemolytic

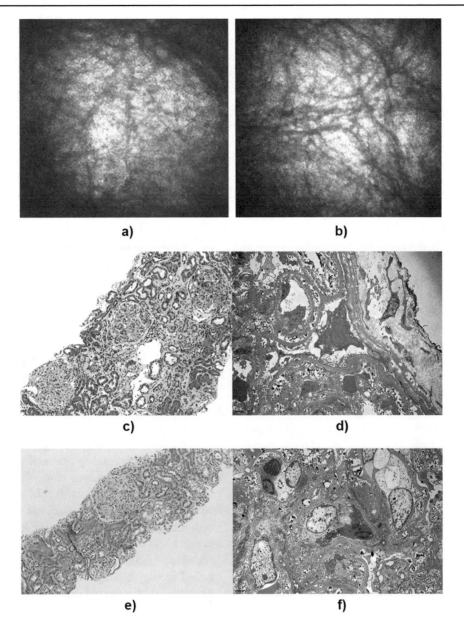

Fig. 3 (**a**, **b**) Multiple dark striae and diffuse hyperreflectivity; (**c**) Enlargement of the mesangium, slightly thickened GBM and foci of interstitial fibrosis with atrophic tubules (LM, by haematoxylin and eosin stain (HES) 100×); (**d**) Deposits of heterogeneous electrondense lipid material were located on the subendothelial side of the GBM and in the mesangium (EM, 4,000×); (**e**) Thickening and double contour of the capillary walls of the glomeruli, with vacuolated mesangial matrix (LM, HES 100×); (**f**) Subendothelial, intramembranous and mesangial heterogeneous electrondense lipid material, surrounded by an electro-lucent zone (EM, 4,000×)

anaemia are not typical of FLD and instead suggest an attenuated phenotype. Moreover, the normal serum ratio of free to esterified cholesterol observed in the proband is indicative of a significant level of residual LCAT activity. The mild, nonspecific intellectual disability manifested by his brother is not attributable to the enzyme deficiency (Santamarina-Fojo et al. 2001).

In vivo confocal microscopy demonstrated the presence of the characteristic corneal opacities in LCAT deficiency: multiple dark striae and hyperreflective deposits diffusely present throughout the stroma, corresponding to excessive extracellular deposition of cholesterol. These findings allow the differential diagnosis with other metabolic corneal dystrophies (Palmiero et al. 2009).

Persistence of unconjugated hyperbilirubinemia despite the complete recovery of anaemia observed in both patients after kidney transplantation, and the lack of any biochemical or haematological markers of chronic haemolysis, led us to consider the differential diagnosis of Gilbert syndrome. This was indeed confirmed by molecular analysis of the 5′

promoter region of UGT1A1, as the two sibs were found to carry the most common genotype associated with Gilbert syndrome in the Caucasian population.

Thrombocytopenia was the only haematological abnormality that did not correct after kidney transplantation and, in the absence of hypersplenism or bone marrow abnormalities, its cause remained elusive. Although thrombocytopenia is not a feature of the classical phenotype of FLD, it has been reported in association with partial deficiency of plasma LCAT activity, in a boy with a peculiar disease phenotype (De Buyzere et al. 1992), without noticeable corneal involvement up to the age of 20 years.

On LM examination of kidney biopsies of FLD patients, the typical presentation is a glomerulopathy with prominent accumulation of lipid-containing, vacuolated foam cells in capillaries and the mesangium (Hirashio et al. 2014). The mesangial matrix is often expanded, and segmental sclerosis is present in more advanced cases. The glomerular basement membrane (GBM) is thickened, with segmental areas of vacuolated appearance; on silver-stained sections, GBM resembles late-stage membranous nephropathy (Hirashio et al. 2014). Unfortunately, the proband's native kidney biopsy was not examined by electron microscopy (EM), and the paraffin-embedded fragments were no longer available for review. However, as it is quite unlikely that the striking glomerular foam cell infiltrate characteristic of FLD was overlooked on the original LM examination, we hypothesize that in patients with residual LCAT activity and kidney involvement, the major histopathological feature might be a membranous nephropathy. This is in line with the report of a patient presenting with nephrotic syndrome caused by immune-mediated acquired LCAT deficiency (Takahashi et al. 2013), whose baseline kidney biopsy exhibited glomerular lesions similar to those of FLD, together with changes of membranous nephropathy. A follow-up kidney biopsy, obtained 5 months after the initiation of steroids and clinical improvement with serum LCAT activity normalization, showed a marked reduction in the glomerular foam cells, and improvement of the mesangial lesions, but persistence of diffuse GBM thickening.

Lp-X stimulates monocyte infiltration of the glomeruli via a mechanism involving mesangial monocyte chemoattractant protein-1 (MCP-1/CCL2) expression (Lynn et al. 2001). The upregulation of MCP-1 mRNA expression and the increased activity of the proinflammatory nuclear factor kappa B (NF-κB) transcription factor in mesangial cells suggest that Lp-X induces inflammatory response in those cells (Lynn et al. 2001). In the LCAT knockout mouse model, only those in which Lp-X was detected developed proteinuria and glomerulosclerosis (Lambert et al. 2001).

Therefore, the immunosuppressive and anti-inflammatory actions of steroids, including the repression of the activity of NF-κB, might antagonize the proinflammatory action of Lp-X in glomerular cells and the pathogenesis of the FLD nephropathy. Combined treatment with nicotinic acid and fenofibrate has been reported to decrease plasma Lp-X levels and the urine albumin/creatinine ratio in a patient with FLD (Yee et al. 2009). In a report of a patient with FLD followed-up for 5 years, lipid-lowering drugs and angiotensin II receptor blockers showed benefit in blood pressure, lipid profile, proteinuria and kidney function (Aranda et al. 2008).

The role of LCAT in the development of atherosclerosis and cardiovascular disease remains incompletely understood. The paradoxical low atherosclerotic risk in LCAT deficiency (Calabresi et al. 2005, 2009), particularly in FDL, has been partly explained by kinetic studies that demonstrated an increased catabolism of LDL and by an up-regulation of the LDL receptor pathway (Nishiwaki et al. 2006).

Currently, there is no specific treatment available for LCAT deficiency but the infusion of recombinant human LCAT (rhLCAT) into mouse models of LCAT deficiency rapidly restored the normal lipoprotein phenotype in LCAT-KO mice and increased cholesterol efflux, suggesting that it might be used as an enzyme replacement therapy (ERT) agent for LCAT deficiency (Rousset et al. 2010). Furthermore, incubation of plasma obtained from FLD subjects and from healthy controls with rhLCAT led to normalization of the lipid/lipoprotein profile in the former, while no major changes were observed in the latter (Simonelli et al. 2013).

A phase 1b, open-label, single-dose escalation study of rhLCAT therapy in subjects with stable CHD and low HDL demonstrated favourable, dose-dependent pharmacodynamic effects on HDL metabolism, with acceptable safety and tolerability (Shamburek et al. 2016a, b). Also encouraging were the beneficial changes in clinical, biochemical and lipoprotein parameters observed in a single patient with FLD and advanced CKD, during an 8-month course of ERT, supporting continued development of rhLCAT therapy (Shamburek et al. 2016a, b) and highlighting the role of Lp-X as a possible biomarker for its monitoring (Shamburek et al. 2016a, b).

Whether rhLCAT therapy is effective to halt CKD progression if started at an earlier stage of the disease will have to be carefully assessed in future clinical trials. Until then, and since ESRD is the major cause of morbidity and mortality in patients with FLD (Myhre et al. 1977), renoprotective therapy by optimal control of blood pressure and reduction of proteinuria using drugs acting on the

RAAS should be instituted as soon as the diagnosis of FLD is established. Although anecdotal evidence (Miarka et al. 2011) suggests that corticosteroid treatment may delay the progression of the FLD-associated nephropathy in the native kidneys, its recurrence in the allograft has been consistently reported in kidney-transplanted FLD patients (Panescu et al. 1997; Strom et al. 2011; Hui Liew et al. 2016), even though corticosteroids are standard therapy in kidney transplantation.

In conclusion, we describe an incomplete clinical and biochemical FLD phenotype, followed by histologically confirmed recurrence of the primary kidney disease in the renal allograft, in two sibs who are most probably homozygous for a novel LCAT missense variant. The atypical phenotype, the delayed recognition and semiological valuing of the corneal opacification, the coexistence of Gilbert syndrome, the diagnosis of membranous nephropathy in the proband's native kidney biopsy, as well as late allograft recurrence of the primary disease, all contributed to obscure the diagnosis of an LCAT deficiency syndrome for many years.

A major teaching point is that on standard LM examination the kidney biopsies of patients with LCAT deficiency and residual enzyme activity, presenting with nephrotic proteinuria and CKD, may not show significant vacuolization and may be misdiagnosed as membranous nephropathy. The cases of these two patients also illustrate the importance of performing detailed physical examination in young adults presenting with proteinuric CKD, as the most important clue to the diagnosis of FLD is in the eyes (Kettritz et al. 2009). Pending the availability of ERT, the mainstay of treatment is intensive blood pressure control and minimization of proteinuria, using RAAS blocking drugs.

Acknowledgements We thank the patients and their mother and older sister for having participated in this study and consented to its publication.

The LCAT gene mutational analysis of the proband was performed at GENDIA (GENetic DIAgnostic Network; http://www.gendia.net/), purchased as an outsource laboratory service.

The UGT1A1 promoter sequence analysis was performed at the "Instituto de Genética Médica Jacinto Magalhães" (Porto, Portugal), purchased as an outsource laboratory service.

Take Home Message

LCAT deficiency diagnosis may be misleading, particularly in atypical phenotypes, highlighting the importance of a detailed physical examination in patients presenting with proteinuric CKD, as the most important clue to the diagnosis of FLD is in the eyes.

Details of the Contributions of Individual Authors

Dr. Inês Castro Ferreira	provided clinical data and drafted the manuscript;
Dr. Rute Carmo	performed the kidney biopsy and drafted the manuscript;
Dr. Sérgio Estrela Silva	performed the ophthalmological examinations and provided clinical data and the relevant photographs;
Dr. Otília Corrêa	performed the lipid and lipoprotein analyses;
Dr. Susana Fernandes	performed the LCAT genetic analysis and provided the electropherogram;
Dr. Susana Sampaio	performed histopathological evaluation of kidney allograft biopsies and provided the relevant illustrations/ photographs;
Dr. Pedro Rodrigues Pereira	performed histopathological evaluation of kidney allograft biopsies and provided the relevant illustrations/ photographs;
Dr. Augusta Praça	provided clinical data;
Prof. Dr. João Paulo Oliveira	provided clinical data and drafted the manuscript and is the guarantor for the chapter.

Corresponding Author

I. Castro-Ferreira.
E-mail: inescastroferreira@sapo.pt.

Details of Funding

None.

Compliance with Ethics Guidelines

Conflict of Interest

Inês Castro Ferreira, Rute Carmo, Sérgio Estrela Silva, Otília Corrêa, Susana Fernandes, Susana Sampaio, Pedro Rodrigues Pereira, Augusta Praça and João Paulo Oliveira declare that they have no conflict of interest.

Informed Consent

All procedures followed were in accordance with the ethical standards of the responsible committee on human experimentation (institutional and national) and with the Helsinki Declaration of 1975, as revised in 2000. Informed consent was obtained from all patients for being included in the study.

Ethical Standards

There are no identifiable patient's personal data on this manuscript.

The publication of this manuscript was approved by the Committee on Ethics for Health of the Centro Hospitalar São João/Faculdade de Medicina da Universidade do Porto.

Reference

Aranda P, Valdivielso P, Pisciotta L et al (2008) Therapeutic management of a new case of LCAT deficiency with a multifactorial long-term approach based on high doses of angiotensin II receptor blockers (ARBs). Clin Nephrol 69:213–218

Calabresi L, Pisciotta L, Costantin A et al (2005) The molecular basis of lecithin-cholesterol acyltransferase deficiency syndromes: a comprehensive study of molecular and biochemical findings in 13 unrelated Italian families. Arterioscler Thromb Vasc Biol 25:1972–1978

Calabresi L, Baldassarre D, Castelnuovo S et al (2009) Functional lecithin-cholesterol acyltransferase is not required for efficient atheroprotection in humans. Circulation 120:628–635

Charlton-Menys V, Pisciotta L, Durrington PN et al (2007) Molecular characterization of two patients with severe LCAT deficiency. Nephrol Dial Transplant 22:2379–2382

De Buyzere M, Delanghe J, Labeur C et al (1992) Acquired hypolipoproteinemia. Clin Chem 38:776–781

Hirashio S, Ueno T, Naito T, Masaki T (2014) Characteristic kidney pathology, gene abnormality and treatments in LCAT deficiency. Clin Exp Nephrol 18:189–193

Kettritz R, Elitok S, Koepke ML, Kuchenbecker J, Schneider W, Luft FC (2009) The case: the eyes have it! Kidney Int 76:465–466

Kuivenhoven JA, Pritchard H, Hill J et al (1997) The molecular pathology of lecithin-cholesterol acyltransferase (LCAT) deficiency syndromes. J Lipid Res 38:191–205

Kunnen S, Van Eck M (2012) Lecithin-cholesterol acyltransferase: old friend or foe in atherosclerosis? J Lipid Res 53:1783–1799

Lambert G, Sakai N, Vaisman BL et al (2001) Analysis of glomerulosclerosis and atherosclerosis in lecithin-cholesterol acyltransferase deficient mice. J Biol Chem 276:15090–15098

Liew H, Simpson I, Kanellis J, Mulley WR (2016) Recurrent glomerulopathy in a renal allograft due to lecithin-cholesterol acyltransferase deficiency. Nephrology (Carlton) 21(1):73–74

Lynn EG, Siow YL, Frohlich J, Cheung GT, O K (2001) Lipoprotein-X stimulates monocyte chemoattractant protein-1 expression in mesangial cells via nuclear factor-kappa B. Kidney Int 60:520–532

Miarka P, Idzior-Waluœ B, KuŸniewski M, Waluœ-Miarka M, Klupa T, Sułowicz W (2011) Corticosteroid treatment of kidney disease in a patient with familial lecithin-cholesterol acyltransferase deficiency. Clin Exp Nephrol 15:424–429

Myhre E, Gjone E, Flatmark A, Hovig T (1977) Renal failure in familial lecithin-cholesterol acyltransferase deficiency. Nephron 18:239–248

Nishiwaki M, Ikewaki K, Bader G et al (2006) Human lecithin-cholesterol acyltransferase deficiency: in vivo kinetics of low-density lipoprotein and lipoprotein-X. Arterioscler Thromb Vasc Biol 26:1370–1375

Ossoli A, Neufeld EB, Thacker SG et al (2016) Lipoprotein X causes renal disease in LCAT deficiency. PLoS One 11(2):e0150083

Palmiero P-M, Sbeity Z, Liebmann J, Ritch R (2009) In vivo imaging of the cornea in a patient with lecithin-cholesterol acyltransferase deficiency. Cornea 29:1061–1064

Panescu V, Grignon Y, Hestin D et al (1997) Recurrence of lecithin-cholesterol acyltransferase deficiency after kidney transplantation. Nephrol Dial Transplant 12:2430–2432

Rousset X, Vaisman B, Auerbach B et al (2010) Effect of recombinant human lecithin-cholesterol acyltransferase infusion on lipoprotein metabolism in mice. J Pharmacol Exp Ther 335(1):140–148

Santamarina-Fojo S, Hoeg J, Assmann G, Brewer HBJ (2001) Lecithin-cholesterol acyltransferase deficiency and fish eye disease. In: Scriver CR, Beaudet AL, Sly WS, Valle D (eds) The metabolic and molecular bases of inherited disease. McGraw-Hill, New York, pp 2817–2833

Shamburek RD, Bakker-Arkema R, Auerbach BJ et al (2016a) Familial lecithin-cholesterol acyltransferase deficiency: first-in-human treatment with enzyme replacement. J Clin Lipidol 10 (2):356–367

Shamburek RD, Bakker-Arkema R, Shamburek AM et al (2016b) Safety and tolerability of ACP-501, a recombinant human lecithin-cholesterol acyltransferase, in a phase 1 single-dose escalation study. Circ Res 118(1):73–82

Simonelli S, Tinti C, Salvini L et al (2013) Recombinant human LCAT normalizes plasma lipoprotein profile in LCAT deficiency. Biologicals 41:446–449

Skretting G, Blomhoff JP, Solheim J, Prydz H (1992) The genetic defect of the original Norwegian lecithin-cholesterol acyltransferase deficiency families. FEBS Lett 309:307–310

Strom EH, Sund S, Reier-Nilsen M, Dorje C, Leren TP (2011) Lecithin-cholesterol acyltransferase (LCAT) deficiency: renal lesions with early graft recurrence. Ultrastruct Pathol 35:139–145

Takahashi S, Hiromura K, Tsukida M et al (2013) Nephrotic syndrome caused by immune-mediated acquired LCAT deficiency. J Am Soc Nephrol 24:1305–1312

Yee MS, Pavitt DV, Richmond W et al (2009) Changes in lipoprotein profile and urinary albumin excretion in familial LCAT deficiency with lipid lowering therapy. Atherosclerosis 205:528–532

JIMD Reports
DOI 10.1007/8904_2017_59

RESEARCH REPORT

Mitochondrial 3-Hydroxy-3-Methylglutaryl-CoA Synthase Deficiency: Unique Presenting Laboratory Values and a Review of Biochemical and Clinical Features

**Erin Conboy · Filippo Vairo · Matthew Schultz ·
Katherine Agre · Ross Ridsdale · David Deyle ·
Devin Oglesbee · Dimitar Gavrilov · Eric W. Klee ·
Brendan Lanpher**

Received: 23 June 2017 / Revised: 28 August 2017 / Accepted: 29 August 2017 / Published online: 14 October 2017
© Society for the Study of Inborn Errors of Metabolism (SSIEM) 2017

Abstract We report an 8-month-old infant with decreased consciousness after a febrile episode and reduced oral intake. He was profoundly acidotic but his lactate was normal. Serum triglycerides were markedly elevated and HDL cholesterol was very low. The urine organic acid analysis during the acute episode revealed a complex pattern of relative hypoketotic dicarboxylic aciduria, suggestive of a potential fatty acid oxidation disorder. MRI showed extensive brain abnormalities concerning for a primary energy deficiency. Whole exome sequencing revealed heterozygotic *HMGCS2* variants. *HMGCS2* encodes mitochondrial 3-hydroxy-3-methylglutaryl-CoA (HMG-CoA) synthase-2 (*HMGCS2*), which catalyzes the irreversible and rate-limiting reaction of ketogenesis in the mitochondrial matrix. Autosomal recessive HMG-CoA synthase deficiency (HMGCS2D) is characterized by hypoketotic hypoglycemia, vomiting, lethargy, and hepatomegaly after periods of prolonged fasting or illness. A retrospective analysis of the urine organic acid analysis identified 4-hydrox-6-methyl-2-pyrone, a recently reported putative biomarker of HMGCS2D. There was also a relative elevation of plasma acetylcarnitine as previously reported in one case. Our patient highlights a unique presentation of HMGCS2D caused by novel variants in *HMGCS2*. This is the first report of HMGCS2D with a significantly elevated triglyceride level and decreased HDL cholesterol level at presentation. Given this, we suggest that HMGCS2D should be considered in the differential diagnosis when hypertriglyceridemia, or low HDL cholesterol levels are seen in a child who presents with acidosis, mild ketosis, and mental status changes after illness or prolonged fasting. Although HMGCS2D is a rare disorder with nonspecific symptoms, with the advent of next-generation sequencing, and the recognition of novel biochemical biomarkers, the incidence of this condition may become better understood.

Communicated by: Jörn Oliver Sass

Erin Conboy and Filippo Vairo contributed equally to this work.

E. Conboy · K. Agre · D. Deyle · D. Oglesbee · D. Gavrilov ·
B. Lanpher
Department of Clinical Genomics, Mayo Clinic, Rochester, MN, USA

E. Conboy · F. Vairo · K. Agre · D. Deyle · D. Gavrilov · E.W. Klee ·
B. Lanpher (✉)
Center for Individualized Medicine, Mayo Clinic, Rochester, MN,
USA
e-mail: Lanpher.Brendan@mayo.edu

M. Schultz · R. Ridsdale · D. Oglesbee · D. Gavrilov
Department of Laboratory Medicine, Mayo Clinic, Rochester, MN,
USA

Introduction

Mitochondrial 3-hydroxy-3-methylglutaryl-CoA (HMG-CoA) synthase is a 471-residue, 51,350-Da peptide that catalyzes the irreversible and rate-limiting reaction of ketogenesis within the mitochondrial matrix. *HMGCS2* maps to chromosome 1p12–13. *HMGCS2* encodes for the mitochondrial HMG-CoA synthase which is highly abundant in the liver in contrast to a cytoplasmic form of HMG-CoA synthase, which is encoded by a homologous *HMGCS1*, and is targeted to the cytoplasm. Through a proposed three-step reaction, HMG-CoA synthase mediates the formation of HMG-CoA, a required intermediate of ketone bodies and a precursor of mevalonate and cholesterol (Mitchell et al. 2014). Ketone bodies are necessary for energy transfer, particularly to the brain, during periods of fasting.

HMG-CoA synthase deficiency (MIM: 605911; HMGCS2D) is a rare autosomal recessive inborn error of metabolism that presents in the first year of life with hypoketotic hypoglycemia, vomiting, lethargy, and hepatomegaly after a period of prolonged fasting or intercurrent illness (Morris et al. 1998; Thompson et al. 1997; Ramos et al. 2013). Some cases have reported acidosis in addition to these symptoms (Morris et al. 1998). Diagnosis of HMGCS2D is problematic, but it can be made using molecular genetic testing or by enzyme activity measurement (Ramos et al. 2013). More recently, the phenotypic spectrum has expanded as children have been identified with HMGCS2D after periods of hypoglycemia during early childhood (Pitt et al. 2015).

We describe an 8-month-old infant who presented with encephalopathy, hepatomegaly, Kussmaul breathing, and high anion gap metabolic acidosis. Uniquely, this child had a markedly elevated triglyceride level with very low high-density lipoproteins (HDL) cholesterol, a finding not yet observed in previously published cases of HMGCS2D.

Materials and Methods

IRB and Patient Consent

We evaluated the proband at the Mayo Clinic in Rochester, MN, USA, with parental consent. The study protocol was approved by the Mayo Clinic Institutional Review Board.

Biochemical Testing

Biochemical testing was performed at the Mayo Clinic Biochemical Genetics Laboratory. Urine organic acids were analyzed by gas chromatography-mass spectrometric analysis of trimethylsilyl ethers of urinary organic acids as previously described (Rinaldo 2008). Plasma acylcarnitines were analyzed by tandem mass spectrometry of butylated carnitine esters as previously published (Rinaldo et al. 2008). Figures and reference ranges for acetylcarnitine analysis were established from 24,671 normal profiles with the aid of Collaborative Laboratory Integrated Reports (CLIR) software.

Genetic Analysis

Whole exome sequencing (WES) of the proband was performed at the Baylor Miraca Genetics Laboratory (Houston, Texas, USA). In summary, for the paired-end pre-capture library procedure, genome DNA is fragmented by sonicating genomic DNA and ligating to the Illumina multiplexing PE adapters. The adapter-ligated DNA is then PCR amplified using primers with sequencing barcodes. For target enrichment/exome capture procedure, the pre-capture library is enriched by hybridizing to biotin labeled VCRome 2.1 in-solution exome probes at 47°C for 64–72 h. Additional probes for over 3,600 Mendelian disease genes were also included in the capture in order to improve the exome coverage. For massively parallel sequencing, the post-capture library DNA is subjected to sequence analysis on Illumina HiSeq platform for 100 bp paired-end reads. The following quality control metrics of the sequencing data are generally achieved: >70% of reads, aligned to target, >95% target base covered at 20×, >85% target base covered of target bases >100×. SNP concordance to genotype array: >99%. The individual's DNA was also analyzed by an SNP array (Illumina HumanExome-12v1 array). The output data from Illumina HiSeq were converted from blc file to FASTQ file by Illumina CASAVA 1.8 software and mapped by BWA program to the Genome Reference Consortium human genome build 37. The variant calls and annotations were performed using algorithms developed in-house by the laboratory. Sanger sequencing was performed in the proband's and parents' DNA for variant confirmation. The *HMGCS2* cDNA reference sequence used was NM_005518.3.

Results

Patient Case

At presentation, the patient was 8-month-old male born at term after an uncomplicated pregnancy and delivery to non-consanguineous parents. There were no perinatal concerns. State newborn screening was normal. His growth, development, and health were normal prior to presentation. He presented after several days of upper respiratory illness symptoms and decreased oral intake. He became unresponsive after a febrile episode and emesis. A rapid Kussmaul breathing pattern was noted. Laboratory investigations in the emergency department revealed an initial metabolic acidosis with pH of 6.8, and subsequently a pH of 7.0 with an anion gap of −28. Urinary dipstick showed ketones at 40 mg/dL (reference: negative), a point of care lactate was normal at 0.79 (reference: 0.6–2.3 mmol/L), and glucose was normal at 3.89 mmol/L (reference range: 3.89–5.55 mmol/L). He received intravenous fluids prior to labs being obtained. His AST and ALT was elevated at 686 and 161 U/L (reference range: AST 8–60 U/L, ALT: 7–55 U/L). Total cholesterol was within normal limits at 4.06 mmol/L, but his triglycerides were significantly elevated at 18.84 mmol/L (reference range: cholesterol: normal <4.4 mmol/L, triglycerides: normal <1.7 mmol/L) and returned to normal ranges when checked 1 week after presentation. Non-HDL cholesterol was 3.98 mmol/L; HDL cholesterol was 0.07 mmol/L (reference range for non-HDL cholesterol is not well established in children, HDL cholesterol normal >0.9 mmol/L). He also had significant thrombocytopenia with platelet counts as low as 10×10^9/L (reference range: 150–450 $\times 10^9$/L). No other similarly affected family members, including 3-year-old sister were reported.

An abdominal ultrasound revealed hepatomegaly with increased echogenicity and coarse echotexture. New onset seizures began while the patient was hospitalized. A brain MRI showed extensive abnormalities of signal, diffusion, and perfusion throughout the gray and white matter (Fig. 1a). MR spectroscopy of the right basal ganglia, parietal white matter, and cerebellum reveals diffusely decreased NAA:choline ratios with large lactate peaks at 1.35 ppm, and amino acid/macromolecular peaks at 0.9 ppm. Increased glutamate-glutamine peaks at 2.1–2.5 and 3.75 ppm, and mildly depleted myoinositol peaks at 3.56 ppm, suggesting a primary energy failure with neurotoxic by-products and disrupted cerebral autoregulation. There was also evidence of cerebral venous congestion and soft tissue edema. Electroencephalography showed multiple and multifocal discharges consistent with status epilepticus. Five-month follow-up MRI showed significant volume loss as well as extensive white matter encephalomalacia (Fig. 1b).

At 15 months of age, the proband continued to be profoundly delayed, without the ability to sit or stand independently, with significant head lag, lack of consistent visual tracking, and intractable seizures. He is gastrostomy-tube-dependent. Despite the resolution of his acute metabolic decompensation, we expect that the severity of brain injury will have a significant impact on his cognitive and physical development.

Biochemical Testing

Urine organic acid analysis during an acute episode revealed a complex pattern of metabolites. Ketone bodies (3-hydroxy-*n*-butyric acid and acetoacetic acid) as well as lactic acid were detected at moderate amounts. The excretion of adipic acid was markedly elevated (539 mmol/mol creatinine; reference: <15), while other dicarboxylic acids were increased to a lesser extent or in the normal range, including suberic (24 mmol/mol; reference: <8) and sebacic acid (1 mmol/mol; reference: <8). Glutaric acid excretion was markedly elevated (557 mmol/mol creatinine; reference: <13) with a moderate amount of 3-OH glutaric acid. Acylcarnitine testing did not detect an elevation of glutarylcarnitine (C5-DC) in the plasma or urine, a result inconsistent with glutaric acidemia type I. The origin of glutaric acid in his urine sample is unclear and possibly related to impaired ketogenesis. 4-hydroxyphenyl lactate and 4-hydroxyphenyl pyruvate were also elevated in a typical tyrosyluria pattern consistent with liver injury. Several unusual trans-hydroxyhexenoic acids were present at moderate concentrations and not components of a typical organic acid profile (Fig. 2a). Two days after presentation, the glutaric acid remained mildly elevated (23 μmol/mmol creatinine) as well as a minimal lactic aciduria and resolving tyrosyluria. These abnormalities normalized in urine over a number of days with dextrose infusion and nutritional support.

Initial plasma acylcarnitine analysis did not demonstrate abnormalities consistent with a recognized disorder of fatty

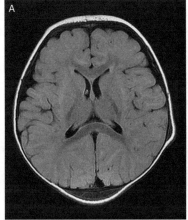 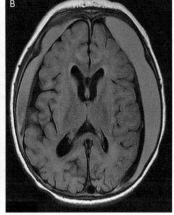

Fig. 1 T2/FLAIR axial view MRI showing (**a**) multifocal hyperintense signal abnormality involving the cerebral cortex, subcortical white matter, and basal ganglia at presentation. (**b**) Five months later, images showing development of moderate bihemispheric cerebral volume loss with involvement of both gray and white matter. Extensive white matter encephalomalacia with progressive, now-confluent hypointense signal throughout the subcortical white matter, preferentially involving arcuate fibers

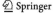

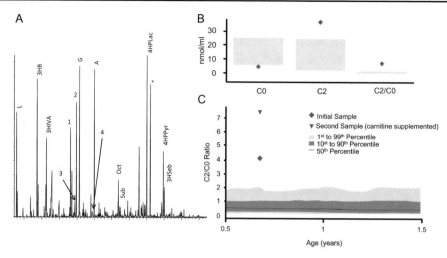

Fig. 2 Biochemical testing. (**a**) Organic acid profile during acute episode. Metabolites identified in Pitt et al. (2015) are numbered (*1* Trans-3-OH-Hex-4-enoic acid, *2* Trans-5-OH-Hex-2-enoic acid, *3* 3,5 adipic lactone, *4* 4-hydroxy-6-methyl-2-pyrone). Relevant metabolites are identified (*L* lactic, *3HB* 3-hydroxy-*n*-butyric, *3HIVA* 3-hydroxyisovaleric, *G* glutaric, *A* adipic, *Oct* octenendioc, *Sub* suberic, *4HPLac* 4-hydroxyphenyllactate, *4HPyr* 4-hydroxyphenyl-pyruvic, *3HSeb* 3-hydroxysebacic). (**b**) Patient's C0, C2, and C2/C0 values after carnitine supplementation during his acute episode. (**c**) His C2/C0 ratio before and after carnitine supplementation during his acute episode compared to reference samples

acid oxidation or organic acidemia. He was found to be carnitine deficient with a decreased free carnitine fraction of 4 nmol/mL and acylcarnitine fraction of 23 nmol/mL. He was subsequently supplemented with L-carnitine at a dose of 100 mg/kg three times daily. A repeat sample taken after supplementation revealed an acetylcarnitine (C2) concentration (37 nmol/mL; reference percentiles: 1st percentile = 2.14, 50th percentile = 6.25, 99th percentile = 21.87), which was relatively elevated compared to other acylcarnitine species in the profile (Fig. 2b). His acylcarnitine testing beyond this acute episode was unremarkable. Initial plasma amino acid analysis showed a nonspecific pattern, most notably with elevations in branched chain amino acids consistent with prolonged fasting.

Molecular Genetic Testing

Given the strong suspicion that this child had an inborn error of metabolism, rapid whole-exome sequencing with concurrent mitochondrial DNA analysis revealed compound heterozygous variants in *HMGCS2*. A maternally inherited, pathogenic variant leading to a stop codon at c.409A>T (p.Lys137*) was observed alongside another variant of uncertain significance, c.1141A>G (p. Met381Val), which was paternally inherited. The proband's sister harbored only the maternally inherited variant c.409A>T (p.K137*). The variant, c.409A>T (p. Lys137*), was not observed in approximately 6,500 individuals of European or African American ancestry as cataloged by the NHLBI Exome Sequencing Project (ESP), or from over 60,000 participants of the Exome Aggregation

Consortium (ExAC). The other missense variant, c.1141A>G (p.Met381Val), was not seen in ESP or ExAC. In silico prediction algorithms resulted in conflicting predictions and that estimated the variant as either tolerable, possibly damaging, disease causing, or possibly pathogenic (SIFT (Kumar et al. 2009), PolyPhen-2 (Adzhubei et al. 2010), Mutation-Taster2 (Schwarz et al. 2014), and M-CAP (Jagadeesh et al. 2016), respectively). Based on the very low allele frequency, compound heterozygosity with a pathogenic variant, residue evolutionary conservation, and biochemical results, this novel variant was classified as likely pathogenic via American College of Medical Genetics and Genomics (ACMG) variant classification guidelines (Richards et al. 2015). Sanger sequencing confirmed both variants in the proband and his parents. Other family members beyond his sister, who was a carrier for the c.409A>T variation, were untested at present time. Mitochondrial DNA analysis was insignificant. Worth noting, *GCDH* which mutations cause glutaric aciduria type 1 had a good coverage on WES and no variants were found.

Discussion

HMGCS2D is an autosomal recessive inborn error of metabolism typically presenting within the first year of life after a period of prolonged fasting and illness. Symptoms include hypoketotic hypoglycemia, vomiting, lethargy, and hepatomegaly (Pitt et al. 2015). Prior reports note increased liver echogenicity suggestive of fatty infiltrate as well as abnormal liver function, as seen in our patient (Wolf et al. 2003). Free fatty acid elevations were previously reported in patients with HMGCS2D during a metabolic crisis (Zschocke et al. 2002). Although this laboratory value was unchecked in our patient while ill, he did present with significantly elevated triglycerides which normalized after 3 days of intensive care. HMGCS2D impairs ketogenesis through an inefficient conversion of fatty acids to ketones. This ketogenesis deficiency, as well as hypoglycemia, may lead to increased lipolysis and marked elevation of free fatty acids as well as, likely, triglycerides (Fukao et al. 2014). A clinical and biochemical comparison between all reported patients with HMGCS2D is seen in Table 1.

Our patient's urine organic acid profile is similar to those previously reported (Zschocke et al. 2002; Aledo et al. 2001), however the profile differed in several key aspects. The dicarboxylic aciduria was composed of primarily adipic acid, while suberic and sebacic acid were only minimally or insignificantly elevated. In addition, glutaric acid excretion was markedly elevated and was not a component described in previous organic acid profiles. Ketone bodies were present in moderate amounts as observed by others for HMGCS2D (Fukao et al. 2014). HMG-CoA can be formed through the catabolism of leucine which may account for the observed ketones. Additionally, this analysis could not distinguish the isomers of 3-hydroxy-*n*-butyric acid, and thus, we cannot confirm that the profile consists of only the D-isomer of 3-hydroxybutyrate. Upon retrospective analysis, the proposed disease-specific metabolites reported by Pitt et al. (2015) were detected in this patient's organic acid profile. Trans-3-hydroxyhex-4-enoic and trans-5-hydroxyhex-2-enoic acids were prominent metabolites in the initial profile while 3,5-dihydroxylhexenoic-1,5-lactones and 4-hydroxy-6-methyl-

Table 1 Comparison of the biochemical and clinical features of the reported individuals with *HMGCS2* deficiency

	This report	Thompson et al. (1997)	Morris et al. (1998)	Aledo et al. (2001)	Zschocke et al. (2002)	Wolf et al. (2003)	Aledo et al. (2006)	Ramos et al. (2013)	Pitt et al. (2015)
Number of patients	1	1	1	1	1	2	2	1	8
Youngest presentation of symptoms	8 months	6 years	16 months	11 months	9 months	19 months	7 months	15 months	5 months
Biochemical features (present in at least one patient)									
Elevated ammonia	−	?	?	?	−	−	?	?	+
Elevated lactate	+	?	−	−	−	−	−	?	+
Elevated free fatty acids	?	+	+	+	+	+	+	+	+
Elevated triglycerides	+	?	?	?		?	?	?	?
Low HDL	+	?	?	?		?	?	?	?
Ketosis	+	−	−	−	−	−	−	+	−
Dicarboxylic aciduria	+	−	+	+	+	+	+	+	+
Elevated C2 after carnitine supplementation	+	?	?	?	?	?	+	?	−
Clinical and other laboratory features (present in at least one patient)									
Decompensation after illness	+	+	+	+	+	+	+	+	+
Hypoketotic hypoglycemia	−	+	+	+	+	+	+	+	+
Coma	+	+	+	+	+	+	+	?	+
Hepatomegaly	+	+	+	+	+	+	+	+	+
Elevated liver function testing	+	+	+	+	−	+	+	+	+
Improvement of metabolic disturbance after intravenous glucose administration	+	+	+	−	+	+	+	+	+

+ present, − absent, ? unknown

2-pyrone were detected in minimal amount only (Fig. 2a). While the presence of these metabolites may point towards a putative HMGCS2D diagnosis, in our experience, these metabolites are present in other conditions including long chain hydroxy acyl-CoA dehydrogenase deficiency and severe ketosis (unpublished observations). This case strengthens the recommendation that the presence of these metabolites in the urine during the setting of acute hypoglycemic episode should prompt investigation for HMG-CoA synthase deficiency by molecular or enzymatic methods.

Upon reexamination of the plasma acylcarnitine profiles around our patient's acute episode, we noted a relative elevation of acetylcarnitine (C2) during his episode (Fig. 2b), which may reflect the same biochemical findings reported by Aledo et al. (2001). In that report, a marked increase in acetylcarnitine was observed after supplementing a decompensated HMG-CoA synthase deficient patient with intravenous L-carnitine. They hypothesized that a buildup of acetyl-CoA combined with carnitine deficiency during an episode of decompensation resulted in an elevated acetylcarnitine concentration upon carnitine supplementation. In our patient's testing, acetylcarnitine was in the normal range at presentation but elevated after supplementation. While the value obtained after supplementation is not elevated to the extent seen in Aledo et al., our case represents the second description of an elevated acetylcarnitine value after L-carnitine supplementation during an acute decompensation.

Noting a relative increase in acetylcarnitine in the setting of carnitine deficiency, we investigated whether an acetylcarnitine/free carnitine (C2/C0) ratio could be a possible clue to the biochemical diagnosis of HMGCS2D. The patient's C2/C0 ratio was elevated at presentation (Ratio = 4.2; reference percentiles: 1st percentile = 0.22, 50th percentile = 0.5, and 99th percentile = 1.83), resulting from a low free carnitine value (4.1 nmol/mL; reference percentiles: 1st percentile = 5.46, 50th percentile = 12.85, 99th percentile = 24.21) and an acetylcarnitine value in the normal range (C2 = 17.2 nmol/mL; reference percentiles: 1st percentile = 2.14, 50th percentile = 6.25, 99th percentile = 21.87). In subsequent acylcarnitine testing 8 h post carnitine supplementation the C2/C0 ratio was further elevated (Ratio = 7.5) resulting from an increase in C2 (37.0 nmol/mL) and relatively unchanged C0 (4.9 nmol/mL) (Fig. 2c). In our experience, these C2/C0 ratio values are elevated even compared to known patient profiles of fatty acid oxidation disorders and organic acidemias (not shown). Similar C2/C0 ratio values are observed in physiologic ketosis; however, this

possibility can quickly be excluded clinical by large excretion of ketone bodies. We propose that an elevated C2/C0 ratio in the absence of significant ketosis during an episode of acute hypoglycemia is an additional biochemical signature of HMGCS2D. This observation will need further study to identify whether there is sufficient specificity for clinical utilization.

The MRI changes seen in our patient characterized by "lentiform fork" sign of metabolic acidosis, with branching linear diffusion abnormality surrounding the basal ganglia along bilateral external capsules, external capsules, and medullary laminae could be secondary to undocumented hypoglycemia, since brain abnormalities are not major features of HMGCS2D per se.

Importantly, our case represents a phenotypic expansion on the biochemical profile of cases previously reported. In particular, our case is the first to be reported with a significantly elevated triglyceride level and decreased HDL cholesterol upon presentation. HMGCS2D certainly leads to a relative depletion of HMG-CoA, but the relationship between this and the low HDL cholesterol and high triglyceride level is not apparent. Further delineation of this mechanism will require studying additional affected patients.

Conclusion

This report highlights a unique presentation of HMGCS2D caused by novel compound heterozygous variants in *HMGCS2* identified by whole-exome sequencing. HMGCS2D is a rare disorder that is believed to be underdiagnosed as the symptoms are often nonspecific and may be mistaken for other metabolic conditions (Aledo et al. 2006). However, with the advent of next-generation sequencing, the incidence of this condition may become better understood. Additionally, this diagnosis should be considered when an individual presents with coma induced by fasting, with hypertriglyceridemia, an elevated C2/C0 ratio, or a low HDL cholesterol level from the newborn period through childhood.

Acknowledgement The authors would like to thank the patient, his family, and the Mayo Clinic Center for Individualized Medicine team for support.

Synopsis

3-Hydroxy-3-methylglutaryl-CoA (HMG-CoA) synthase-2 deficiency is a rare disorder with a specific urine organic acid profile, and recently found to have presenting laboratory abnormalities of hypertriglyceridemia and low HDL.

Details of the Contributions of Individual Authors

Erin Conboy, Filippo Vairo, Matthew Schultz: Contributed significantly to the manuscript and critically reviewed manuscript.

Brendan Lanpher, David Deyle, Katherine Agre: Saw patient and critically reviewed, contributed to the manuscript, and edited manuscript.

Ross Ridsdale, Devin Oglesbee, Dimitar Gavrilov: Were essential in the analysis and interpretation of the molecular and biochemical lab results, contributed to the intellectual content of the manuscript and critically reviewed and edited manuscript.

Eric W. Klee: Was essential in the variant interpretation for the Whole-Exome Data, contributed to the intellectual content of the manuscript, and critically reviewed and edited manuscript.

Conflicts of Interest

The authors have no conflicts of interest or competing interests pertaining to the manuscript.

No funding sources were required for this work.

The study protocol was approved by the Mayo Clinic Institutional Review Board.

The patient and family consented to this report.

No laboratory animals were used for this work.

References

Adzhubei IA et al (2010) A method and server for predicting damaging missense mutations. Nat Methods 7(4):248–249

Aledo R et al (2001) Genetic basis of mitochondrial HMG-CoA synthase deficiency. Hum Genet 109(1):19–23

Aledo R et al (2006) Refining the diagnosis of mitochondrial HMG-CoA synthase deficiency. J Inherit Metab Dis 29(1):207–211

Fukao T et al (2014) Ketone body metabolism and its defects. J Inherit Metab Dis 37(4):541–551

Jagadeesh KA et al (2016) M-CAP eliminates a majority of variants of uncertain significance in clinical exomes at high sensitivity. Nat Genet 48(12):1581–1586

Kumar P, Henikoff S, Ng PC (2009) Predicting the effects of coding non-synonymous variants on protein function using the SIFT algorithm. Nat Protoc 4(7):1073–1081

Mitchell GA, Fukao T (2014) Inborn errors of ketone body metabolism. In: Beaudet AL et al (eds) The online metabolic and molecular bases of inherited disease. McGraw-Hill, New York

Morris AA et al (1998) Hepatic mitochondrial 3-hydroxy-3-methylglutaryl-coenzyme a synthase deficiency. Pediatr Res 44(3):392–396

Pitt JJ et al (2015) Mitochondrial 3-hydroxy-3-methylglutaryl-CoA synthase deficiency: urinary organic acid profiles and expanded spectrum of mutations. J Inherit Metab Dis 38(3):459–466

Ramos M et al (2013) New case of mitochondrial HMG-CoA synthase deficiency. Functional analysis of eight mutations. Eur J Med Genet 56(8):411–415

Richards S et al (2015) Standards and guidelines for the interpretation of sequence variants: a joint consensus recommendation of the American College of Medical Genetics and Genomics and the Association for Molecular Pathology. Genet Med 17(5):405–424

Rinaldo P (2008) Organic acids. In: Duran M, Blau N, Gibson KM (eds) Laboratory guide to the methods in biochemical genetics. Springer, Berlin, pp 137–170

Rinaldo P, Cowan TM, Matern D (2008) Acylcarnitine profile analysis. Genet Med 10(2):151–156

Schwarz JM et al (2014) MutationTaster2: mutation prediction for the deep-sequencing age. Nat Methods 11(4):361–362

Thompson GN et al (1997) Fasting hypoketotic coma in a child with deficiency of mitochondrial 3-hydroxy-3-methylglutaryl-CoA synthase. N Engl J Med 337(17):1203–1207

Wolf NI et al (2003) Mitochondrial HMG-CoA synthase deficiency: identification of two further patients carrying two novel mutations. Eur J Pediatr 162(4):279–280

Zschocke J et al (2002) The diagnosis of mitochondrial HMG-CoA synthase deficiency. J Pediatr 140(6):778–780

JIMD Reports
DOI 10.1007/8904_2017_63

RESEARCH REPORT

Extended Experience of Lower Dose Sapropterin in Irish Adults with Mild Phenylketonuria

S. Doyle · M. O'Regan · C. Stenson · J. Bracken ·
U. Hendroff · A. Agasarova · D. Deverell · E. P. Treacy

Received: 04 May 2017 / Revised: 16 September 2017 / Accepted: 20 September 2017 / Published online: 14 October 2017
© Society for the Study of Inborn Errors of Metabolism (SSIEM) 2017

Abstract Adherence to dietary and treatment recommendations is a long-standing concern for adults and adolescents with PKU and treating clinicians. In about 20–30% of PKU patients, Phe levels may be controlled by tetrahydrobiopterin (BH4) therapy. The European PKU 2017 Guidelines recommends treatment with BH4 for cases of proven long-term BH4 responsiveness, with a recommended dosage of Sapropterin 10–20 mg/kg/day.

We report four young Irish patients with mild PKU, known to be BH4 responsive, who were treated with lower doses of Sapropterin for over 7 years.

Case 1: Female, currently age 20. Genotype p. I65T/p/ F39L, c.[194T>C]; [117C>G]. Newborn Phe: 851 μmol/L. Pre-Sapropterin Phe tolerance: 600 mg Phe/day to maintain Phe levels <400 μmol/L. Commenced on Sapropterin 400 mg (6.5 mg/kg/day) with increase in Phe tolerance to 800 mg/day.

Case 2: Female, currently age 23. Genotype p. I65T/ pF39L; c.[194T>C]; [117C>G]. Newborn Phe: 714 μmol/L. Pre-Sapropterin Phe tolerance: 700 mg Phe/day. Commenced on Sapropterin 400 mg (8 mg/kg/day) with increase in Phe tolerance to 800 mg/day.

Case 3: Male, currently age 22. Genotype p. I65T/p. S349P; c.[194T>C][1045T>C]. Newborn Phe: 1,036 μmol/ L. Pre-Sapropterin Phe tolerance: 600 mg Phe/day. Commenced on Sapropterin 400 mg (5.4 mg/kg/day). Increased to 1,600 mg Phe/day.

Case 4: Female, currently age 29. Genotype p.R408W/p/ p.Y414C; c.[1222C>T], [1241A>G]. Newborn Phe: 1,600 μmol/L. Pre-Sapropterin tolerance: 450 mg/day. Commenced on Sapropterin 400 mg (5.0 mg/kg/day). Increased to 900 mg Phe/day.

Almost 7 years of surveillance for these four patients has shown that this dose of Sapropterin (range 5–8 mg/kg day) was well tolerated and effective with a significant response to treatment and a marked improvement in quality of life at these lower Sapropterin doses.

Background

Adherence to dietary control and treatment recommendations is a long-standing concern to clinicians involved with the care of adult and adolescent PKU patients. In a recent US survey of 182 clinics, it was noted that >60% of adolescents (age 13–17) and >70% of adult PKU patients attending US clinics are non-adherent to target phenylalanine concentrations consistent with earlier international reports (Jurecki et al. 2017; Walter et al. 2002). This is evidenced by non-attendance at clinic and inadequate blood monitoring. Poor adherence leads to social difficulties, mood disorders, attention difficulties and executive functioning difficulties (Burton et al. 2013; Arnold et al. 2004). Patients frequently report poor palatability of the protein substitutes which leads to poor compliance. Furthermore,

Communicated by: Avihu Boneh, MD, PhD, FRACP

S. Doyle · J. Bracken · U. Hendroff · A. Agasarova · E.P. Treacy (✉)
National Centre for Inherited Metabolic Disorders, The Mater
Misericordiae University Hospital, Dublin, Ireland
e-mail: etreacy@mater.ie

S. Doyle · E.P. Treacy
University College Dublin, Dublin, Ireland

M. O'Regan · C. Stenson · E.P. Treacy
National Centre for Inherited Metabolic Disorders, The Children's
University Hospital, Dublin, Ireland

D. Deverell
Department of Pathology, The Children's University Hospital, Dublin,
Ireland

patients report a negative impact of Phenylketonuria (PKU) and its management on their life with high levels of anxiety concerning high phenylalanine levels (Bosch et al. 2015). Pregnancy represents additional challenges in managing PKU with high anxiety reported among expectant mothers (Bosch et al. 2015).

However, recent European guidelines for the treatment and management of patients with PKU advises a 'treatment for life' approach for PKU. For patients over age 12, an upper Phe target of 600 μmol/L is recommended to aim to maintain optimum outcomes and neuropsychological functioning (Van Spronsen et al. 2017). The American College of Genetics and Genomics (Vockley et al. 2014) recommends an upper target Phe concentration of 360 μmol/L for adults with PKU.

At least 890 mutations are now described at the *PAH* locus (BioPKU database, https://www.biopku.org). In about 20–30% of PKU patients, Phe levels may be controlled by tetrahydrobiopterin therapy (Heintz et al. 2013). Sapropterin dihydrochloride is a synthetic formulation of Tetrahydrobiopterin (BH4), a naturally occurring essential cofactor for PAH that acts as a pharmacological chaperone and decreases blood phenylalanine levels and increases dietary phenylalanine tolerance in a subset of patients with milder PKU with BH4 responsive genotypes (Hennermann et al. 2012; Lindegren et al. 2013; Scala et al. 2015).

According to the European PKU Guidelines, treatment with BH4 should only be prescribed in cases of proven long-term BH4 responsiveness defined as the increase in amount of natural protein tolerated of 100% or more or with improved biochemical control (Phe levels >75% in target range) and proven by a trial of up to 6 months. The recommended dosage of Sapropterin is 10–20 mg/kg/day body weight (Van Spronsen et al. 2017). In this case report we retrospectively report our experience with four adult patients with Sapropterin responsive mild PKU treated with lower dose Sapropterin (5–8 mg/kg/day).

Methods

Four Irish patients with mild PKU who were known to be BH4 responsive were treated with lower doses of Sapropterin (BH4) since 2010. Two of these patients (subject numbers 2 and 4) had entered the initial 6 week randomised placebo controlled study of Sapropterin and continued in the 22 week extension study using forced dose titrations of 5, 20 and 10 mg/kg/day (Levy et al. 2007; Lee et al. 2008). The four patients (young adults), one male and three female, had genotypes known to be BH4 responsive (see Table 1). This report outlines their response to treatment as measured by their average Phe level, the amount of natural protein consumed daily as recently assessed, the required intake of synthetic protein, their self-reported improvement in quality of life on BH4 based on a structured interview and a recent evaluation using the adult version of the PKU specific Health-related Quality of Life (HRQoL) questionnaire. The PKU HRQoL questionnaire specifically assesses the impact of PKU on all aspects of PKU patients' lives, including PKU symptoms; the practical social and emotional impact of the condition, the impact of low-protein dietary restrictions and the impact of Phe-free amino acid supplements. Scores of <25% indicate little or no impact of the disease, scores of >25 and <50% indicate a moderate impact, scores of >50 and <75% indicate a major impact and scores of >75% indicate severe impact (Bosch et al. 2015).

Dietary information was collated from a retrospective review of dietetic records for each patient. The current dietary intake was a 'typical day' recall from each patient's last dietetic OPD visit, taken within the past 6 months. Anthropometric measurements and micronutrient status assessment (including ferritin, B12, folate, Hb, and Zn and Se where indicated) were measured before and after Sapropterin use and at each clinic visit.

Table 1 Description of four patients with PKU, biochemical characterisation/Phe tolerance

Case Number and Gender	1 (F)	2 (F)	3 (M)	4 (F)
Newborn Phe level (μmol/L)	851	714	1,036	1,600
Genotype	165T/F39L	165T/F39L	165T/S349P	R408W/Y414C
Pre-Sapropterin Phe tolerance (mg)	600	700	600	450
Recent Phe tolerance (mg)	800	800	1,600	900
Current Sapropterin dose (mg/kg/day)	6.25	8.0	5.4	5
Length of time on Sapropterin (years)	7	7	7	7
Synthetic protein intake g/day. Pre-Sapropterin and post-Sapropterin (in brackets)	60 (40)	50 (42)	60 (40)	75 (50)
Mean (median) Phe level for last 5 years on treatment (μmol/L)	394 (386)	548 (539)	602 (568)	510 (506)
Phe range (min–max) μmol/L	96–868	201–926	287–1,108	345–690

A dietetic phone questionnaire was conducted with each subject by a qualified dietitian based on a list of common questions/topics. Questions included in the interview addressed how the PKU diet was perceived to be different after the use of Sapropterin; how many exchanges were allowed in the diet before and after Sapropterin; the changes in synthetic protein required; and the changes in intake of low protein foods. In addition, questions were formulated as to how these changes affected the individual's lifestyle: such as the ease of food preparation; the ability to eat out at restaurants; the ease of travel; the ease of socialising; and whether taking Sapropterin had proven to be a positive or negative experience.

In addition to this self-reported structured interview, the four subjects completed the adult PKU specific HRQoL questionnaire. It should be noted that this PKU specific quality of life assessment tool has been available since 2015 and was not available for these individuals before they commenced BH4.

Results

Case 1 Female, currently age 20. Genotype p.165T/p. F39L, c.[194T>C]; [117C>G]. The phenylalanine level in the newborn period was 851 μmol/L (Mild PKU). Pre-Sapropterin at age 13, her Phe tolerance was 600 mg Phe/day to maintain phenylalanine levels <400 μmol/L. She was commenced on maintenance 400 mg Sapropterin (6.25 mg/kg/day) in 2010. This individual has self-reported improved quality of life with improved diet palatability and flexibility since commencing Sapropterin.

Case 2 Female, currently age 23. Genotype p.165T/p. F39L; c.[194T>C]; [117C>G]. The phenylalanine level in the newborn period was 714 μmol/L (mild PKU). Pre-Sapropterin Phe tolerance was 700 mg Phe at age 7. Commenced on Sapropterin 400 mg (8 mg/kg/day) in 2010. This individual reports an ease of meal preparation since starting the treatment facilitating preparation of her own meals which were previously prepared by her parents. She also described increased freedom and choice in relation to food choices resulting in less anxiety around meals.

Case 3 Male, currently age 22. Genotype p165T/p.S349P; c.[194T>C][1045T>C]. The phenylalanine level in the newborn period was 1,036 μmol/L (mild PKU). Pre-Sapropterin Phe tolerance was 600 mg. Commenced on Sapropterin 400 mg (5.4 mg/kg/day) in 2010. This individual reports that he can now eat out with friends more often allowing for improved social life which was

important to him. He also described previously hiding his synthetic drinks which is less of an issue now. He feels the treatment has been 'life changing' and allowed him to live a 'normal life'.

Case 4 Female, currently age 29. Genotype: p.R408W/p. Y414C; c.[1222C>T], [1241A>G]. Phenylalanine level in the newborn period was 1,600 μmol/L (mild PKU). Pre-Sapropterin Phe tolerance was 450 mg/day. Commenced on Sapropterin 400 mg (5.0 mg/kg/day) in 2010. This individual is now enjoying eating out which she feels was not possible before starting the treatment due to the restricted diet.

For subjects 2 and 4, these individuals had previously participated in the Sapropterin Phase III extension study (Lee et al. 2008). Thus, they were commenced on a starting dose of 5 mg/kg/day Sapropterin based on the previously identified response at this dose. The phenylalanine levels were measured on a weekly basis and the natural protein exchanges were increased weekly in increments from 100 to 200 mg phenylalanine while maintaining plasma phenylalanine levels <400 μmol/L.

For subject 2, the phenylalanine intake was increased by 100 mg per week to 1,000 mg after 2 months. This individual has had difficulties with recurrent urinary tract infections and subsequently the phenylalanine intake was stabilised at 800 mg/day (Table 1). The initial synthetic protein requirement for subject 2 was 50 g/day which subsequently was decreased to 30 g/day and in recent years to 42 g/day.

Initially, during the first 6 months of Sapropterin, subject 4 tolerated an increase of phenylalanine of 350 mg/day phenylalanine with an increase to 450 mg over the last 2 years. The synthetic protein daily requirement was decreased from 75 to 50 g.

Subjects 1 and 3 had not previously been enrolled in the Sapropterin trial but were known to have BH4 potentially responsive mutations. Both patients initially were started on Sapropterin 10 mg/kg/day for 1 week which determined responsiveness, and then continued on 5 mg/kg/day for 6 weeks as an initial trial period. Subject 1 increased the phenylalanine daily intake from 600 mg phenylalanine/day to 1,000 mg/day initially, then stabilising to 800 mg/day over time. Her synthetic protein intake was reduced from 60 to 40 g/day.

For subject 3, the patient tolerated an increase in phenylalanine by approximately 200 mg/week, from 600 to 2,000 mg/day, then subsequently stabilised on 1,600 mg/day. His synthetic protein requirement and intake decreased from 60 to 40 g/day.

According to the patient's weight, the dose was subsequently rounded for all patients to 400 mg or 500 mg/day (Table 1).

On serial yearly blood monitoring of micronutrient status, two cases required intervention: (Subject 2 and 4) during the last 4 years of treatment. Subject 2 manifested a transient B12 deficiency (154 nmol/L) associated with poor adherence to the prescribed vitamin and mineral supplement in tablet form. Adherence improved with education. Subject 4 manifested chronic sub-optimal zinc levels associated with intermittent reduced intake of the prescribed amino acid supplement and minimal dietary sources of zinc, despite an increase in her natural protein allowance. The zinc status improved after this patient was prescribed additional multi-vitamins to provide an additional 20–40% per day of her vitamin and mineral requirements to ensure ongoing adequacy of her diet.

The above examples highlight the need for ongoing micronutrient monitoring with changes in the dietary prescription associated with a change to Sapropterin. However, it should be noted that poor adherence to intake of the amino acid supplement was well documented in both these individuals prior to starting Sapropterin and indeed was a major rationale to start this therapy.

Height, weight and BMI were monitored and recorded at each OPD visit. In the past 4 years there has been minimal fluctuation in BMI for each patient. Cases 1–3 started Sapropterin in adolescence and therefore earlier BMI records will require interpretation using BMI centile charts and are not included here. Case 4 started therapy in adulthood and has maintained a similar BMI throughout the past 7 years.

The mean phenylalanine levels over the previous 5 years of treatment for all four patients while on Sapropterin are illustrated in Table 1 with the pre-treatment levels, genotype, Sapropterin dose, current natural protein tolerance, changes in synthetic protein intake/requirement and recent PKU HRQoL assessments (Table 2) for three of the four subjects. Other than very occasional high Phe levels with intercurrent illness, the four subjects obtained excellent biochemical control on treatment (Table 1).

The Quality of Life as self-reported by all four subjects was noted to be improved post treatment with Sapropterin. All respondents indicated that travel was now much easier without having the necessity to bring vast amounts of low protein foods and all respondents recommended the treatment and reported that it had a positive impact on their lives. The PKU HRQoL domains studied for the three individuals all noted little or no current impact of the disease. Table 2 shows the results for all four domains for the three respondents that answered the questionnaire.

From a review of the most recent dietary record taken in out-patients and a patient phone questionnaire, all four individuals reported improved variety in regular foods they are able to consume and less reliance on specialised low protein prescription foods such as bread, pasta, biscuits, flours, milks. This involved the use of normal bread/wraps, chips and pasta/noodles and increased flexibility of choices, for example toppings on pizzas, ability to eat out at restaurants and to take small quantities of higher protein foods such as meat on occasion for subjects 2 and 3.

Discussion

Almost 7 years of surveillance for these four patients has shown that this dose of Sapropterin (range 5–8 mg/kg day) was well tolerated and effective. There were no adverse effects noted and all four subjects reported a marked improvement of their Quality of Life with optimum Phe levels and adherence during this time period. All four subjects considered that the liberalised diet possible as a result of Sapropterin treatment had a positive impact on their life.

The literature cites differing experiences with Quality of Life assessments in PKU patients that are shown to be responsive to Sapropterin. In a US based study, Douglas

Table 2 PKU health-related quality of life score under domain and categorisation

Quality of Life (QoL) score under domain (%) followed by category	Case 1	Case 2	Case 3	Case 4
Symptoms	4% Minimum impact QoL	0 No impact QoL	16% Little or no impact QoL	25% Little or no impact QoL
Adherence	20% Little or no impact QoL	4.5% Little or no impact QoL	7.6% Little or no impact QoL	29% Moderate impact on QoL
Supplement use (synthetic formula and products)	15% Little or no impact QoL	20% Little or no impact QoL	12.5% Little or no impact QoL	25% Little or no impact QoL
Protein restriction	15.5% Little or no impact QoL	4.8% Little or no impact QoL	6.25% Little or no impact QoL	21.5% Little or no impact QoL

et al. (2013) reported significant improved Quality of Life (QoL) for definitive Sapropterin PKU responders in their study (17 BH4 responders). The areas of improvement noted by the patients described in this report include: reduced planning required for meals, more freedom around eating out allowing more socialising, and increased independence around food preparation. Cazzoria et al. (2014) reported the experience of 22 Italian PKU patients with mild PKU who were respondent to BH4 in comparison to 21 patients with classical PKU treated with diet. Global QoL scores were found to be within the normal range both in patients with mild and classical PKU but global QoL was found to be significantly higher in patients with mild PKU under BH4 treatment as compared to the classical PKU group under a complete dietary Phe restriction regime (Cazzoria et al. 2014). In the study reported by Demirdas et al. (2013) of Dutch patents attending eight metabolic centres, overall PKU patients demonstrated normal health-related quality of life (HRQoL), however for the 10 BH4 responsive PKU patients in their study, improvement in their HRQoL after relaxation of diet could not be demonstrated (Demirdas et al. 2013). A recent study by Feldmann et al. (2017) reporting on 112 German BH4 patients (children and adolescents) with PKU measured the QoL for the patients and their carers before the start of BH4 therapy and after 6 months of therapy. This group reported that Sapropterin did not seem to improve the QoL in PKU patients and their carers.

In our current study, three of the four patients showed a significant response to treatment at these lower Sapropterin doses with reduced requirement for synthetic protein and reduced costs associated with using low protein products and self-reported improved quality of life. However, the economic benefit of this improvement of quality of life is difficult to quantify. Ireland is one of the few countries worldwide that has an explicit cost-effectiveness threshold (O'Mahony and Coughlan 2016). In Ireland generally only medicines that are more expensive than existing treatments for similar patients undergo a Health Technology Assessment (HTA) that measures Quality of Life adjusted years (QALYs) with other economic evaluations. A QALY is: 'A measure of an individual's length of life that has been adjusted for the health-related quality of life'. Essentially a QALY equates to 1 year of good health. Quality of Life is measured by quality of life questionnaires. This assessment is challenging for diseases which are not life-threatening when there are alternative treatments (such as dietary in PKU).

While Sapropterin at a dose of 10 mg/kg day has not to date received reimbursement approval in Ireland by the HTA assessment process, we consider that this lower dose schedule may represent a more cost-effective treatment for patients with responsive mutations, allowing a less restrictive diet with improved Quality of Life and improved adherence.

Acknowledgement Ms. Maebh Durkin R. D. is thanked for her assistance with the dietary analysis.

References

Arnold GL, Vladutiu CJ, Orlaski CC et al (2004) Prevalence of stimulant use for attentional dysfunction in children with phenylketonuria. J Inherit Metab Dis 27:137–143

Bosch AM, Burlina A, Cunningham A et al (2015) Assessment of the impact of phenylketonuria and its treatment on quality of life of patients and parents from seven European countries. Orphanet J Rare Dis 10:80. https://doi.org/10.1186/s 13023-015-0294-x

Burton BK, Leviton L, Vespa H et al (2013) A diversified approach for PKU treatment: routine screening yields high incidence of psychiatric distress in phenylketonuria clinics. Mol Genet Metab 108:8–12

Cazzoria C, Cegolon L, Burlina AP et al (2014) Quality of Life (QoL) assessment in a cohort of patients with phenylketonuria. BMC Public Health 14:1243

Demirdas S, Maurice-Stam H, Boelen CC et al (2013) Evaluation of quality of life in PKU before and after introducing tetrahydrobiopterin (BH4); a prospective multi-center cohort study. Mol Genet Metab 110(Suppl):S49–S56

Douglas TD, Ramakrishan U, Kabie JA et al (2013) Longitudinal quality of life analysis in a phenylketonuria cohort provided sapropterin dihydrochloride. Health Qual Life Outcomes 11:218

Feldmann R, Wolfgart E, Weglage J et al (2017) Sapropterin treatment does not enhance the health-related quality of life of patients with phenylketonuria and their parents. Acta Paediatr 106:953–958

Heintz C, Cotton RG, Blau N (2013) Tetrahydrobiopterin, its mode of action on phenylalanine hydroxylase, and importance of genotypes for pharmacological therapy of phenylketonuria. Hum Mutat 34(7):927–936

Hennermann JB, Roloff S, Gebauer C et al (2012) Long-term treatment with tetrahydrobiopterin in phenylketonuria: treatment strategies and prediction of long-term responders. Mol Genet Metab 107:294–301

Jurecki ER, Cederbaum S, Kopesky J et al (2017) Adherance to clinic recommendations among patients with phenylketonuria in the United States. Mol Genet Metab 120(3):190–197

Lee P, Treacy EP, Crombez E et al (2008) Safety and efficacy of 22 weeks of treatment with sapropterin dihydrochloride in patients with phenylketonuria. Am J Med Genet 146A(22):2851–2859

Levy HL, Milanowski A, Chakrapani A et al (2007) Efficacy of sapropterin dishydrochloride (tetrahydrobioptern, 6R-BH4) for reduction of phenylanine concentration in patients with phenylketonuria: a phase III randomised placebo-controlled study. Lancet 370(9586):504–510

Lindegren ML, Krishnaswami S, Reimschisel T et al (2013) A systematic review of BH4 (sapropterin) for the adjuvant treatment of phenylketonuria. JIMD Rep 8:109–119

O'Mahony JF, Coughlan D (2016) The Irish cost-effectiveness threshold: does it support rational rationing or might it lead to unintended harm to Ireland's health system? PharmacoEconomics 34(1):5–11

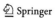

Scala I, Concolino D, Della Casa R et al (2015) Long-term follow-up of patients with Phenylketonuria treated with tetrahydrobiopterin: a seven years experience. Orphanet J Rare Dis 10:14. https://doi.org/10.1186/s13023-015-0227-8

Van Spronsen FJ, Van Wegberg AM, Ahring K et al (2017) Key European guidelines for the diagnosis and management of patients with phenylketonuria. Lancet Diabetes Endocrinol 5 (9):743–756. https://doi.org/10.1016/S2213-8587(16)30320-5. [Epub ahead of print]

Vockley J, Andersson HC, Antshel KM et al (2014) Phenylalanine hydroxylase deficiency: diagnosis and management guideline. Genet Med 16:188–200

Walter JH, White FJ, Hall SK et al (2002) How practical are recommendations for dietary control in phenylketonuria? Lancet 360(9326):55–57

JIMD Reports
DOI 10.1007/8904_2017_65

RESEARCH REPORT

Fumarase Deficiency: A Safe and Potentially Disease Modifying Effect of High Fat/Low Carbohydrate Diet

B. Ryder · F. Moore · A. Mitchell · S. Thompson ·
J. Christodoulou · S. Balasubramaniam

Received: 22 June 2017 / Revised: 24 September 2017 / Accepted: 04 October 2017 / Published online: 21 October 2017
© Society for the Study of Inborn Errors of Metabolism (SSIEM) 2017

Abstract Fumarate hydratase deficiency (FHD) caused by biallelic alterations of the *FH* (fumarate hydratase) gene is a rare disorder of the tricarboxylic acid cycle, classically characterized by encephalopathy, profound psychomotor retardation, seizures, a spectrum of brain abnormalities and early death in childhood. Less common milder phenotypes with moderate cognitive impairment and long-term survival have been reported. In addition, heterozygous mutations of the *FH* gene are responsible for hereditary leiomyomatosis and renal cell cancer (HLRCC). There is currently no recommended disease modifying treatment for FHD and only isolated reports of unsuccessful dietary modifications. Herein, we describe the safe and possibly disease modifying effect of a high fat, low carbohydrate diet in a 14-year-old female with severe FHD.

Communicated by: John H Walter, MD FRCPCH

J. Christodoulou and S. Balasubramaniam contributed equally to this work.

B. Ryder · S. Thompson · J. Christodoulou · S. Balasubramaniam
Western Sydney Genetics Program, The Children's Hospital at Westmead, Sydney, NSW, Australia

F. Moore
NSW Biochemical Genetics Service, The Children's Hospital at Westmead, Sydney, NSW, Australia

A. Mitchell · S. Thompson
Metabolic Dietetic Service, The Children's Hospital at Westmead, Sydney, NSW, Australia

J. Christodoulou · S. Balasubramaniam
Discipline of Genetic Medicine, Sydney Medical School, University of Sydney, Sydney, NSW, Australia

J. Christodoulou · S. Balasubramaniam (✉)
Discipline of Child & Adolescent Health, Sydney Medical School, University of Sydney, Sydney, NSW, Australia
e-mail: saras329@hotmail.com

J. Christodoulou
Neurodevelopmental Genomics Research Group, Murdoch Children's Research Institute, Melbourne, VIC, Australia

J. Christodoulou
Department of Paediatrics, Melbourne Medical School, University of Melbourne, Melbourne, VIC, Australia

Introduction

Fumarate hydratase deficiency, also known as fumarase deficiency, is a rare autosomal recessive disorder of the tricarboxylic acid (TCA) cycle. Fumarate hydratase (FH) (EC 4.2.1.2) catalyses the reversible interconversion of fumarate and malate, and its deficiency leads to impaired energy production due to interruption of the TCA cycle and subsequent accumulation of various TCA intermediates including fumarate, succinate, 2-ketoglutarate and citrate. Fewer than 100 cases have been reported. The highest prevalence of FH deficiency is found in a religious community at the border of northern Arizona and southern Utah, USA, due to a founder effect (Allegri et al. 2010; Kerrigan et al. 2000).

FH deficiency has a varied clinical phenotype ranging from a fulminant course associated with fatal outcome within the first 2 years of life or a subacute encephalopathy with profound developmental delay (Morava and Carrozzo 2014). Acute metabolic crises with hypoglycemia, ketosis, hyperammonemia or acidosis are rarely observed in FH deficiency (Ewbank et al. 2013; Allegri et al. 2010). Antenatal presentations include poly- or oligohydramnios, intrauterine growth retardation, congenital hydrocephalus and other brain abnormalities (Ewbank et al. 2013, Allegri et al. 2010). Severely affected children exhibit progressive infantile encephalopathy, feeding problems, failure to thrive, hypotonia, lethargy, microcephaly, seizures and profound developmental delay. Most severely affected children are usually nonverbal and non-ambulatory. Epileptic seizures are common and are often treatment resistant. Age of onset and seizure type vary and may include infantile spasms with hypsarrhythmia on EEG (Ewbank et al. 2013; Loeffen et al. 2005). Neuroradiological findings include cerebral atrophy, ventriculomegaly, white matter abnormalities including delayed myelination or hypomyelination, thinning or agenesis of the corpus callosum, open opercula, choroid plexus or arachnoid cysts, small brainstem and bilateral diffuse polymicrogyria (Kerrigan et al. 2000). Visual disturbance and optic nerve hypoplasia have occasionally been described (Kerrigan et al. 2000). A spectrum of dysmorphic features has been reported to include common findings of depressed nasal bridge, frontal bossing and widely spaced eyes or less commonly cleft ala nasi or anteverted nares, ear anomalies or narrow forehead (Ewbank et al. 2013; Kerrigan et al. 2000).

Isolated increased concentration of fumaric acid on urine organic acid analysis is highly suggestive of FH deficiency. Other metabolites may also be altered in body fluids: TCA cycle intermediates (succinate, 2-ketoglutarate, citrate), dicarboxylic acids (suberic, adipic) and succinylpurine derivatives (Allegri et al. 2010). Laboratory indicators may include increased lactate, mild hyperammonemia, variable leukopenia, neutropenia and neonatal polycythemia (Allegri et al. 2010). The diagnosis is confirmed by identification of deficient FH enzyme activity in fibroblasts, leukocytes, skeletal muscle or liver and/or by molecular analysis of the *FH* gene (MIM*136850).

There are currently no recognized therapies to ameliorate or reverse the metabolic abnormalities resulting from decreased activity of FH (Morava and Carrozzo 2014). Management remains supportive, with regular multisystem surveillance. We report here a female with fumarase deficiency, predicted to be severe on enzyme and mutational analysis, who has had a milder course, possibly due to early institution of a high fat/low carbohydrate diet.

Case History

The proband was the first-born child to non-consanguineous parents of Italian and Caucasian Australian background. Delivery was by emergency caesarean section at 35 weeks gestation, for maternal hypertension and deranged liver function tests. The pregnancy was otherwise uncomplicated. Birth growth parameters were all above the 90th percentile and Apgar scores were 8 and 9 at 1 and 5 min, respectively. She required tube feeding for the first 4 days, and 24 h of phototherapy for jaundice on day 3. She was discharged on day 10 on a combination of breast and bottle feeds, but continued to have feeding difficulties. By

7 months of age her weight had fallen to the 3rd centile and she was hypotonic with delayed early developmental milestones. A urine metabolic screen at 9 months of age found increased fumaric acid, prompting referral to the metabolic service. On examination at 9 months of age, she had relative macrocephaly with a head circumference on the 75–90th percentile. Her weight was less than the 3rd percentile and length on the 10–25th percentile. She was non-dysmorphic but had eczema and nasal obstruction. She was thin with minimal fat stores and reduced muscle bulk. She was generally hypotonic and unable to sit unsupported. Cardiovascular, respiratory and abdominal examinations were normal. Blood and urine lactates were normal and there were no other urinary tricarboxylic acid cycle (TCA) intermediates present to suggest a mitochondrial disorder. Plasma amino acids and plasma acylcarnitines were normal. The diagnosis was confirmed with cultured skin fibroblast enzyme analysis: fumarate hydratase (FH) activity was 9% of normal controls (patient enzyme activity 9 nmol/min/mg protein, normal reference range 78–119 nmol/min/mg protein) (Mitochondrial Laboratory, Victoria Clinical Genetics Service and Murdoch Children's Research Institute). Molecular analysis revealed compound heterozygous mutations in the *FH* gene (c.521C>G, p.Pro174Arg; c.1204C>T, p.His402Tyr). (Dr V Shih, Neurochemistry Laboratory, Massachusetts General Hospital, Boston MA, USA.) Her parents were found to be heterozygous for one or other of these mutations.

At 14 months of age she was started on a high fat/low carbohydrate diet, with the diet goals of 60% energy from fat, 30% from carbohydrate and 10% from protein. Initiating the diet was complicated by allergy to milk and soy, and increased rate of weight gain (85–97th centile for BMI), but there was a gradual change over the first year from a baseline intake of 36% energy from fat, 48% from carbohydrate and 16% from protein. The diet has been adhered to lifelong with a minimum of 50% fat at times of lesser compliance. She has grown well with close monitoring and dietetic review. Monitored bloods have been generally within normal range, including full blood counts, liver and renal function tests, plasma lactate, plasma amino acids, essential fatty acids, plasma lipids and micronutrient levels. Supplementation of calcium intake has been required. Urine organic acid analysis has never detected lactate or other TCA cycle intermediates and her fumaric acid excretion has reduced to moderate levels. At most recent diet analysis at age 13 years, fat made up 58%, carbohydrate 25% and protein 14%, providing 1.7 g/kg/day protein (RDI 0.87 g/kg). Twenty-two percent of fat was saturated due to dietary preferences and BMI was on the 82nd percentile. Her energy intake was 128% EERM; however, BMI has been consistently been between the 75th and 85th centile since 6 years of age. Her home sick day plan comprises 50:50 lipid:carbohydrate with a target of 2,200 kcal/day (basal EER × 1.2 for illness), and an inpatient emergency plan for illness and surgical procedures advises maintenance intravenous fluids of 0.45% saline with 5% dextrose and 20% intralipid at 2–3 g/kg/day.

Global developmental delay was evident in infancy: she sat unsupported at 11 months, walked at 18 months and had delayed expressive language. Hearing and ophthalmology assessments were normal. A pre-school developmental assessment at 4 years and 7 months found mild to moderate intellectual disability and schooling has been in a special unit. Initial MRI brain at 1 year of age showed mild cerebral atrophy, predominantly affecting the frontal lobes bilaterally. There was a generalised reduction in white matter bulk with prominent lateral ventricles and a slight increase in posterior periventricular white matter signal bilaterally. Myelination was appropriate. The frontal lobe grey matter appearance was suspicious for polymicrogyria. There was onset of seizures with status epilepticus at 22 months of age. Seizures have been relatively well controlled on monotherapy with carbamazepine, apart from a brief period of seizure recurrence in early adolescence of unknown cause. Her most recent EEG at the age of 11 years showed background abnormalities with intermittent slow-ing and bilateral, focal epileptiform discharges without clinical correlation. Serial MRI scans of the brain have shown asymmetrical cerebral sulcal and gyral patterns consistent with polymicrogyria, particularly in the anterior frontal, posterior parietal and temporal lobes. Ventriculo-megaly is thought to reflect parenchymal white matter volume loss (Fig. 1). The Cho/Cr ratio was markedly reduced on MRS in both white matter and basal ganglia; however, the NAA/Cr ratio was normal. No lactate peaks were identified. At age 10 years, she underwent repair of a large multi-fenestrated atrial septal defect with left-to-right shunt and right ventricular dilatation. Consistent with published literature, she has not had any acute metabolic decompensation with illness. Currently, at the age of 14 years she is in a special unit at her school and has a mild-to-moderate intellectual disability. She is an active member of her community and is involved in Girl Guides. She has been seizure free on carbamazepine for more than 1 year and is growing well on the 85th centile for weight, 70th centile for height and 98th centile for head circumfer-ence. Her general health is good, other than hay fever and constipation.

Having reached her teenage years, we have recommen-ded annual abdominal MRI surveillance due to the risk of

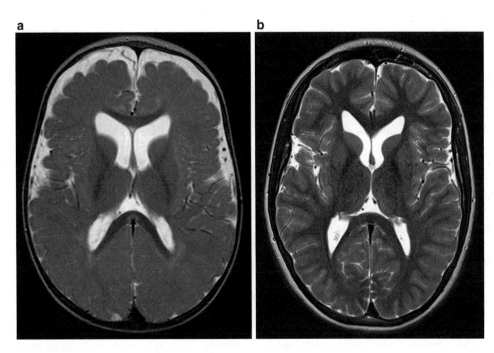

Fig. 1 (**a**) MRI brain aged 12 months. Generalized white matter loss with mild prominence of the ventricular system in keeping with white matter loss. Slight prominence to the grey matter within the mildly atrophied frontal lobes without definite migrational abnormality. (**b**) MRI brain aged 14 years. Asymmetrical mild enlargement of the lateral ventricles likely secondary to parenchymal white mater volume loss. Asymmetrical cerebral sulcal and gyral patterns, particularly of the anterior frontal, posterior parietal and the temporal lobes, are suspicious for polymicrogyria or other cortical malformation

HLRCC and there is, as yet, no evidence of HLRCC. The same screening has been recommended to her parents who have been reviewed by a familial cancer service.

Discussion

Our patient presented before 6 months of age, with typical features of FHD: hypotonia, poor weight gain and developmental delay. Aside from relative macrocephaly there were no overt dysmorphic features. Her MRI findings of diffuse bilateral polymicrogyria, enlarged lateral ventricles and decreased white matter with seizure disorder are characteristic. Her seizure control is much better than reported despite the structural brain abnormalities. Relative macrocephaly has been reported in FHD in association with cerebral atrophy and enlarged extra-axial CSF spaces (Kerrigan et al. 2000). Cardiac involvement in FHD is rare, but ventricular septal defects and patent ductus arteriosus have been reported (Mroch et al. 2012).

A clear genotype–phenotype correlation has not been shown for FHD or HLRCC (Deschauer et al. 2006; Bayley et al. 2008). The FH gene, located at 1q42.1, consists of ten exons encoding 510 amino acids of both mitochondrial and cytosolic isoforms of FH. Most mutations are concentrated at the C-terminus of the FH enzyme (Allegri et al. 2010). There are currently 172 unique variants reported in the Leiden Open Variation Database (LOVD 3.0), many of which are private mutations (http://databases.lovd.nl/shared/genes/FH). Our patient's c.1204C>T (p.His402Tyr) variant in exon 8 has been previously reported in a case of severely affected monozygotic twins, one dying aged 1 year (Phillips et al. 2006). The c.521C>G (p.Pro174Arg) variant in exon 4 has been reported in both HLRCC and severe, fatal FHD (Mroch et al. 2012).

More severe clinical symptoms usually correlate with lower levels of enzyme activity (Ottolenghi et al. 2011), although this relationship has not been clear and consistent in all studies (Morava and Carrozzo 2014). FH enzyme activity less than 10% of the control mean generally results in a severe phenotype (Ottolenghi et al. 2011), although the most profoundly affected individuals have enzyme activity of 1–2% or unrecordable. Residual FH enzyme activity can be 0–35% of the control mean in affected individuals, overlapping with that of obligate heterozygotes (Morava and Carrozzo 2014). Milder cases of FHD are less common and those reported still have moderate developmental delay, often without expressive language (Ezgu et al. 2013; Maradin et al. 2006; Kimonis et al. 2012). A severe phenotype was predicted for our patient based on her presentation with hypotonia and developmental delay by 6 months, her structural brain abnormalities and seizures, and fibroblast enzyme activity 9% of normal controls. In addition, she is compound heterozygous for two mutations previously reported in severe cases with early fatality.

FH functions as a tumour suppressor, rare for an enzyme involved in intermediary metabolism (Bayley et al. 2008). Individuals with germline heterozygous mutations in the FH gene are predisposed to multiple cutaneous and uterine leiomyomas (MCUL) and hereditary leiomyomatosis with renal cell cancer (HLRCC). The gene alteration in HLRCC was identified in 2002 by Tomlinson et al. Pathogenic germline FH mutations have been detected in 76–100% of families with suggestive features (Lehtonen 2011). The estimated lifetime risk of renal cancer in HLRCC is 15% (Menko et al. 2014). Based on the youngest case reported at 10 years of age, predictive FH mutation testing and annual abdominal MRI surveillance with 1–3 mm slices through the kidneys in order to detect very small tumours are recommended from 8 to 10 years of age (Menko et al. 2014). Other syndromic features of cutaneous piloleiomyomas and early uterine fibroids may not be obvious and the aggressive papillary cancers may metastasize when less than 1 cm in diameter (Menko et al. 2014). Renal ultrasound is not recommended due to the low sensitivity in detecting such small lesions. Heterozygote parents of patients with FHD have been reported with HLRCC (Ezgu et al. 2013; Maradin et al. 2006). Early detection is important because of the aggressive nature of renal cancers associated with HLRCC and high death rates of 74% from metastatic disease (Gardie et al. 2011). Treatment should be prompt and generally consists of wide-margin surgical excision and consideration of retroperitoneal lymph node dissection for even small unilateral tumours. The precise risk of HLRCC to individuals affected with FHD is not known, as very few survive to adulthood.

Several mechanisms of tumorigenesis in HLRCC have been proposed. There is decreased oxidative phosphorylation due to disruption of the TCA cycle and impairment of the oxidative function of the electron transport chain. Accumulated fumarate competitively inhibits the function of hypoxia inducible factor (HIF) prolyl hydroxylase (HPH), resulting in HIF accumulation. This in turn leads to an increase in the expression of anti-apoptotic and proliferative genes such as vascular endothelial growth factor (VEGF), platelet-derived growth factor (PGDF) and transforming growth factor-alpha (TGF-alpha), all of which enhance angiogenesis and support tumour growth and survival (Sudarshan et al. 2007; Yang et al. 2012). This in turn results in epigenomic modifications (Xiao et al. 2012).

There are few published reports of dietary interventions in FHD. Fumaric acid is a by-product of protein catabolism; however, a brief therapeutic trial of low protein diet (0.71 g/kg/day for 3 days) proved unsuccessful in altering urinary excretion of fumaric acid or improving clinical signs (Kimonis et al. 2012). Similarly, protein restriction of

0.8 g/kg/day in a 45-day-old infant failed to demonstrate any improvement in the urinary excretion of fumaric acid (Baştuğ et al. 2014). Smith and Robinson used a metabolic model of FHD to assess the ability of various metabolites to increase ATP production in a state of 0% fumarase activity. Supplementation with aspartate appeared most effective in increasing ATP production, perhaps bypassing the enzymatic block by replenishing oxaloacetate (Smith and Robinson 2011). An increase in glucose caused minimal increase in ATP production, but a large increase in lactate. Fatty acid metabolism was reported to be relatively restricted by the block to acetyl CoA entering the TCA cycle, and it has been recommended to avoid the ketogenic diet in FHD (Ewbank et al. 2013).

Contrary to predictions, our patient's clinical progression has followed a milder phenotype with well-controlled seizures and mild-to-moderate intellectual disability, possibly due to the high fat/low carbohydrate dietary intervention commenced at 14 months of age. We propose that a high fat diet may increase the amount of reduced high-energy NADH and $FADH_2$ molecules, allowing adequate ATP generation through the mitochondrial electron transport chain irrespective of reduced TCA cycle activity. As a long chain of reduced carbon atoms, fatty acids fuel more cycles of the TCA cycle than glycolysis, and additionally generate one molecule each of NADH and $FADH_2$, for each cycle of beta-oxidation. Complete beta-oxidation of palmitate requires seven cycles of beta oxidation thereby generating 7 NADH and 7 $FADH_2$ and 8 molecules of acetyl-CoA. Each molecule of acetyl-CoA then releases 2 molecules of NADH and 1 of $FADH_2$, prior to the fumarate block in the TCA cycle (see Fig. 2). Contrary to

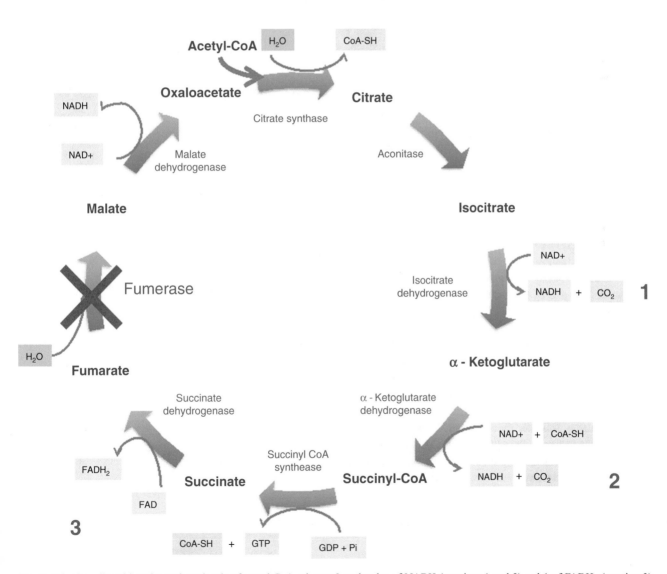

Fig. 2 Tricarboxylic acid cycle: each molecule of acetyl-CoA releases 2 molecules of NADH (reactions 1 and 2) and 1 of $FADH_2$ (reaction 3) prior to the fumarate block in the TCA cycle

Table 1 Semi-quantification of urinary fumaric acid excretion over time

Date	Fumarate (μmol/mmol creatinine)	Comments
24/03/2004	1,262	Diet was commenced in November 2004
21/05/2004	650	
01/06/2004	1,104	
27/06/2005	679	Ketonuria detected in this sample collected during an intercurrent illness
22/11/2016	344	
26/05/2017	429	

Key Synopsis

Long-term use of a high fat, low carbohydrate diet in severe fumarate hydratase deficiency is safe and may result in a milder outcome.

Details of the Contributions of Individual Authors

Bryony Ryder, John Christodoulou and Shanti Balasubramaniam were involved in the clinical management of the patient. Sue Thompson and Ashleigh Mitchell provided dietary advice in the management. Francesca Moore performed and interpreted metabolic laboratory investigations. John Christodoulou advised on the diagnostic work-up and initiating dietary management. Bryony Ryder and Shanti Balasubramaniam drafted the manuscript. All authors have read/critically revised the manuscript.

Smith and Robinson's findings we have not observed a block to fatty acid beta-oxidation.

Our patient has never had elevated plasma or urinary lactate. We propose that a low carbohydrate diet reduces flux through glycolysis, thereby limiting lactate production. We have observed a semi-quantitative reduction in urinary fumaric acid to one-third of levels prior to dietary intervention (see Table 1). Patients with FHD have occasionally been reported with normal urinary fumaric acid excretion (Ottolenghi et al. 2011) and elevations do not correlate reliably with phenotype severity (Prasad et al. 2017). Nonetheless the reduction in her urinary fumarate excretion and the absence of other TCA intermediates may reflect anaplerosis and continuation of the TCA cycle, perhaps through aspartate. Previous attempts at a low protein diet may have reduced anaplerosis. Our patient has not been protein restricted and at last review her protein intake of 1.7 g/kg/day was well above the recommended daily intake for age of 0.87 g/kg/day. Plasma amino acids remain normal.

In summary, our patient had a typical clinical presentation for severe FHD with significant developmental delay by 9 months of age, seizures and structural brain malformations. In addition, her residual fumarase enzyme activity was only 9% of normal and she is compound heterozygous for two mutations previously reported in cases of early fatality. Despite this her development appears to have surpassed any other reported cases of FH. This case is important as it demonstrates after 12 years of follow-up that a high fat/low carbohydrate diet is safe and may be potentially disease modifying.

Acknowledgements No funding was received in the writing of this chapter.

Corresponding Author

Bryony Ryder.

Compliance with Ethics Guidelines

Conflict of Interest

Bryony Ryder, Francesca Moore, Ashleigh Mitchell, Sue Thompson and Shanti Balasubramaniam declare that they have no conflict of interest. John Christodoulou is a communicating editor of the *Journal of Inherited Metabolic Disease*.

Ethics Approval

Ethics approval was not required for publication of this case report.

Informed Consent

Parental consent was obtained for the publication of this chapter.

References

Allegri G, Fernandes MJ, Scalco FB (2010) Fumaric aciduria: an overview and the first Brazilian case report. J Inherit Metab Dis 33(4):411–419

Baştuğ O, Kardaş F, Öztür MA et al (2014) A rare cause of opistotonus; fumaric aciduria: the first case presentation in Turkey. Turk Pediatri Ars 49(1):74–76

Bayley J-P, Launonen V, Tomlinson I (2008) The FH mutation database: an online database of fumarate hydratase mutations involved in the MCUL (HLRCC) tumour syndrome and congenital fumarase deficiency. BMC Med Genet 9(20):1–98

Deschauer M, Gizatullina Z, Schulze A et al (2006) Molecular and biochemical investigations in fumarase deficiency. Mol Genet Metab 88:146–152

Ewbank C, Kerrigan JF, Aleck K (2013) Fumarate hydratase deficiency. In: Pagon RA, Adam MP, Ardinger HH et al (eds) Gene reviews. University of Washington, Seattle

Ezgu F, Pavel K, Wilcox W (2013) Mild clinical presentation and prolonged survival of a patient with fumarase deficiency due to the combination of a known and a novel mutation in FH gene. Gene 524:403–406

Gardie B, Remenieras A, Kattygnarath D (2011) Novel FH mutations in families with hereditary leiomyomatosis and renal cell cancer (HLRCC) and patients with isolated type 2 papillary renal cell carcinoma. J Med Genet 48(4):226–234. http://www.hlrccinfo.org/hlrcc-handbook.php

Kerrigan JF, Aleck KA, Tarby TJ et al (2000) Fumaric aciduria: clinical and imaging features. Ann Neurol 47(5):583–588

Kimonis VE, Steller J, Sahai I et al (2012) Mild fumarase deficiency and trial of a low protein diet. Mol Genet Metab 107(1–2):241–242

Lehtonen HJ (2011) Hereditary leiomyomatosis and renal cell cancer: update on clinical and molecular characteristics. Familial Cancer 10(2):397–411

Loeffen J, Smeets R, Voit T, Hoffmann G, Smeitink J (2005) Fumarase deficiency presenting with periventricular cysts. J Inherit Metab Dis 28(5):799–800

Maradin M, Fumić K, Hansikova H et al (2006) Fumaric aciduria: mild phenotype in an 8-year-old girl with novel mutations. J Inherit Metab Dis 29(5):683

Menko F, Maher ER, Schmidt LS et al (2014) Hereditary leiomyomatosis and renal cell cancer (HLRCC): renal cancer risk, surveillance and treatment. Familial Cancer 13(4):637–644

Morava E, Carrozzo R (2014) Disorders of the Krebs cycle. In: Blau N et al (eds) Physician's guide to the diagnosis, treatment, and follow-up of inherited metabolic diseases. Springer-Verlag, Berlin, pp 313–322

Mroch AR, Laudenschloager M, Flanagan JD (2012) Detection of a novel FH whole gene deletion in the propositus leading to subsequent prenatal diagnosis in a sibship with fumarase deficiency. Am J Med Genet A 158A:155–158

Ottolenghi C, Hubert L, Allanore Y et al (2011) Clinical and biochemical heterogeneity associated with fumarase deficiency. Hum Mutat 32(9):1046–1052

Phillips TM, Gibson JB, Ellison DA (2006) Fumarate hydratase deficiency in monozygotic twins. Pediatr Neurol 35:150–153

Prasad C, Napier P, Rupar C, Prasad C (2017) Fumarase deficiency: a rare disorder on the crossroads of clinical and metabolic genetics, neurology and cancer. Clin Dysmorphol 26:117–120

Smith AC, Robinson AJ (2011) A metabolic model of the mitochondrion and its use in modelling diseases of the tricarboxylic acid cycle. BMC Syst Biol 5:102

Sudarshan S, Linehan WM, Neckers L (2007) HIF and fumarate hydratase in renal cancer. Br J Cancer 96:403–407

Xiao M, Yang H, Xu W et al (2012) Inhibition of α-KG-dependent histone and DNA demethylases by fumarate and succinate that are accumulated in mutations of FH and SDH tumor suppressors. Genes Dev 26(12):1326–1338

Yang M, Soga T, Pollard PJ, Adam J (2012) The emerging role of fumarate as an oncometabolite. Front Oncol 2:85

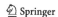

JIMD Reports
DOI 10.1007/8904_2017_66

RESEARCH REPORT

Early Diagnosed and Treated Glutaric Acidemia Type 1 Female Presenting with Subependymal Nodules in Adulthood

Bimal Patel · Surekha Pendyal · Priya S. Kishnani · Marie McDonald · Lauren Bailey

Received: 27 June 2017 / Revised: 06 October 2017 / Accepted: 11 October 2017 / Published online: 01 November 2017
© Society for the Study of Inborn Errors of Metabolism (SSIEM) 2017

Abstract Glutaric acidemia type 1 (GA-1, OMIM no. 231670) is an autosomal recessive disorder caused by the deficiency of glutaryl-CoA dehydrogenase (GCDH). The subsequent accumulation of the amino acids lysine, hydroxylysine, and tryptophan and their breakdown intermediates can be neurotoxic and particularly cause injury to the basal ganglia.

Roughly 1 of 100,000 infants is affected with GA-1, and a common feature at birth is macrocephaly. Stress, such as in febrile illnesses, can precipitate encephalopathic crises in children generally less than 2 years with variable recovery. Many infants develop dystonia with complex movement disorders and subtle cognitive and fine motor deficits. Common neuroradiologic findings include hypoplasia of temporal and frontal lobes, striatal lesions, white matter changes, and subdural effusions.

There are three previous reports of subependymal nodules found on neuroimaging in GA-1 patients who were diagnosed as adults and untreated for GA-1. We present a unique case of an adult female who was diagnosed at age 2 months and managed prior to any metabolic decompensation. Her initial diagnosis was made based on biochemical and enzymatic analysis, and then later confirmed with genetic sequencing. She started experiencing frequent headaches at age 12 years. Neuroimaging in adulthood revealed common features seen in GA-1 in addition to the finding of subependymal nodules.

This case may provide some insight into the natural progression of the disease despite early treatment. Though subependymal nodules are typically seen in tuberous sclerosis, the significance of these lesions in GA-1 is not well understood. Disease courses of more early diagnosed and treated patients with GA-1 need to be documented.

Introduction

Glutaric acidemia type 1 (GA-1, OMIM no. 231670) is an inherited autosomal recessive disorder caused by glutaryl-CoA dehydrogenase (GCDH) deficiency and impairment in the breakdown of amino acids – lysine, hydroxylysine, and tryptophan. The subsequent accumulation of these amino acids and their breakdown intermediates, glutaric acid, glutaryl-CoA, 3-hydroxyglutaric acid, and glutaconic acid, can be neurotoxic and cause striatal injury, affecting the basal ganglia. Also, secondary carnitine deficiency results as a consequence of its consumption in metabolism of glutaric acid.

Roughly 1 of 100,000 infants worldwide is affected and often born with macrocephaly. Stress, such as in dehydration, surgery, reactions to vaccinations, or febrile illnesses, can exacerbate encephalopathic crises in children less than 2 years of age with variable recovery after each episode. Many infants develop dystonia with complex movement disorders and subtle cognitive and fine motor deficits. Commonly documented neuroradiologic findings include hypoplasia of temporal and frontal lobes, striatal lesions, white matter changes, and subdural effusions (Twomey et al. 2003). Though historically this disorder has been

Communicated by: William Ross Wilcox, MD, PhD

B. Patel
Department of Hospital Medicine, Duke University Hospital, Durham, NC, USA

S. Pendyal · P.S. Kishnani (✉) · M. McDonald · L. Bailey
Division of Medical Genetics, Department of Pediatrics, Duke University Hospital, Durham, NC, USA
e-mail: priya.kishnani@duke.edu

associated with the aforementioned central nervous system involvement, recent publications have suggested other organ damage in the peripheral nervous and renal systems (Herskovitz et al. 2013; Kölker et al. 2015).

With the advancement of newborn screening and early diagnosis, initiation of a low lysine diet, carnitine supplementation, and intensified emergency management during catabolism can prevent metabolic crises. There is now expected to be a large number of asymptomatic individuals with GA-1 who have a good prognosis and are followed into adulthood. Though previous recommendations have focused on dietary treatment primarily during the first 6 years of life and relaxed management thereafter, a few documented cases of neuroradiologic abnormalities in adult-onset GA-1 and early treated GA-1 have challenged this prior doctrine (Boy et al. 2017). The natural progression of early diagnosed and treated GA-1 is not fully understood and more case studies need to be documented in the literature. We present a unique case of subependymal nodules found in an adult patient with GA-1 who was diagnosed and treated since infancy without metabolic crises.

Case Report

A Caucasian female first presented with macrocephaly (head circumference-for-age +2.1 standard deviations, Kuczmarski et al. 2000) and megalencephaly at 3 weeks of age. GA-1 was suspected and confirmed through elevated levels of glutaric acid in urine, plasma, and cerebrospinal fluid (CSF) as well as absence of GCDH activity in fibroblasts. Patient has one full sibling, an older brother, without any known symptoms, though he has not had any additional biochemical, enzymatic, or molecular assessments. The family history is significant for some paternal relatives with possible mental retardation and degenerative eye disease. The family is of Northern European descent, primarily German. There is some Native American descent on the maternal side. There are no reported birth defects or consanguinity in the family. The remainder of the family history is otherwise negative for mental retardation, birth defects, multiple pregnancy losses, or known genetic disorders.

No genetic testing was performed initially, but the patient was treated with a low protein diet, carnitine, and riboflavin and closely monitored during intercurrent illnesses. She had otherwise normal neurological presentation and did not have metabolic crises as a child. With treatment and close monitoring, she maintained a sufficient level of executive functioning but did have some learning difficul-

ties in school. As a pre-teenager, she began having headaches. Neurology evaluation at 12 years of age determined her headaches to be migrainous and related to idiopathic intracranial hypertension (IIH) after lumbar puncture (LP) analysis showed high opening pressures.

She graduated from high school but did not attend college. The patient had two successful pregnancies at age 23 and 25 years.

At age 28 years, she presented to the hospital with 3 weeks of slurred speech as well as left facial weakness and numbness. The rest of the exam was normal. Her prior imaging was reviewed. An MRI at age 22 years showed callosal and periventricular white matter changes, age discordant parenchymal atrophy, and multifocal subependymal nodules in the lateral ventricles. These changes were stable on serial imaging at 26 years of age. CT and MRI were repeated during hospital presentation showing no acute changes. LP revealed an opening pressure of 36 cm H_2O, consistent with an exacerbation of IIH. Given her unusual presentation and history of subependymal nodules not previously documented with early diagnosed and treated GA-1, she had genetic testing (*TSC1* and *TSC2* genes) for tuberous sclerosis (TSC) and periventricular nodular hypertopia (*FLNA* gene) which was negative. A CT abdomen at 24 years showed no renal cysts or angiomyolipomas often seen in TSC, and patient had no other stigmata for TSC (such as facial angiofibromas, hypopigmented macules, forehead plaques, or Shagreen patches). Further genetic testing then was done confirming her original biochemical GA-1 diagnosis.

Materials and Methods

Original biochemical and enzymatic diagnosis of GA-1 was performed during infancy. Repeated studies for continued management that also supported her diagnosis included plasma carnitine and acylcarnitines, plasma amino acids, as well as urine organic acids.

Genomic DNA was obtained from fresh blood at 28 years. Genetic testing was then performed using methods applied at a commercial laboratory, GeneDx. The following genes were specifically reviewed with the percentage of the coding region covered at >10X by exome sequencing indicated in parentheses: *FLNA* (100%), *GCDH* (100%), *TSC1* (100%), and *TSC2* (100%). The Agilent Clinical Research Exome kit was used to target the exonic regions and flanking splice junctions. These targeted regions were sequenced simultaneously by massively parallel (NextGen) sequencing on an Illumina HiSeq sequencing system with 100 bp paired-end reads. Bidirectional sequence was assembled, aligned to reference gene sequences based on human genome build GRCh37/UCSC hg19, and analyzed for sequence variants in the selected genes or regions of interest using a custom-developed analysis tool (Xome Analyzer). Capillary sequencing or another appropriate method was used to confirm all potentially pathogenic variants identified in this individual. Sequence alterations were reported according to the Human Genome Variation Society (HGVS) nomenclature guidelines.

Results

At initial presentation as an infant, patient had elevated glutaric acid in plasma, urine, and CSF and absence of GCDH activity in fibroblasts which established the diagnosis of GA-1.

Molecular genetic studies of *FLNA*, *TSC1*, and *TSC2* were normal. However, the patient was found to be homozygous for the c.1204 C>T, p.R402W pathogenic variant in the *GCDH* gene in adulthood confirming her original biochemical diagnosis of GA-1. The homozygous state of the R402W variant of the *GCDH* gene has been reported in multiple patients with clinical features and biochemical profiles consistent with GA-1 (Biery et al. 1996; Busquets et al. 2000; Gupta et al. 2015).

MRI at 29 years showed stable callosal and periventricular white matter changes, age discordant parenchymal atrophy, and multifocal subependymal nodules in the lateral ventricles (Figs. 1 and 2).

Discussion

Subependymal nodules are hamartomatous forms of heterotopia, which are benign yet disorganized growths composed of elements of the adjacent tissue. These lesions line the walls of ventricles and are most common in TSC, infants with TORCH infections, and elderly patients with neoplastic growths of subependymal cells. Subependymal nodules are seen in roughly 80% of patients with TSC. They are thought to be asymptomatic and have no epileptogenic potential. They are of unknown clinical significance, though they are presumed to have theoretical potential to develop into subependymal giant cell astrocytomas, which are the most common brain tumor type in TSC (Klar et al. 2016).

Upon review of the literature, there have been no other cases of GA-1 patients who were early diagnosed and treated since infancy presenting with subependymal nodules. Three cases of subependymal nodules have been reported in patients with GA-1, but all were diagnosed in adulthood and had no other unifying diagnosis (Table 1). All three of these patients had different ethnic backgrounds, presentations, and pathogenic variants in the *GCDH* gene.

Our patient's case reveals that subependymal nodules may develop as a natural progression of GA-1 despite early diagnosis and metabolic control, though their clinical

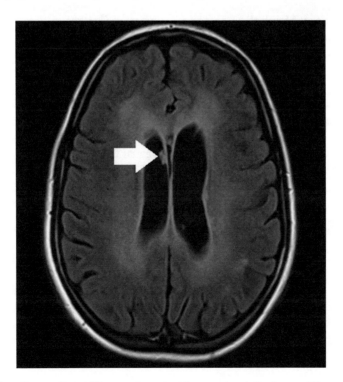

Fig. 1 MRI brain axial flair imaging of case patient at 29 years of age. A white arrow is pointing to one of the periventricular subependymal nodules

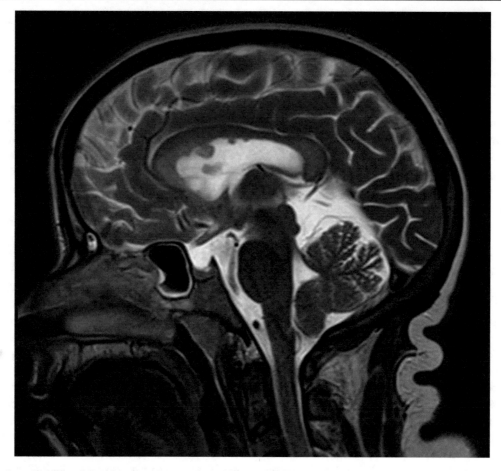

Fig. 2 MRI brain sagittal T2 weighted imaging of case patient at 29 years of age

significance is yet to be determined. More cases needed to be documented in literature.

Synopsis

We report the first case of subependymal nodules in an adult, without any stigmata for tuberous sclerosis, who was diagnosed and treated for glutaric acidemia type 1 since infancy without any metabolic decompensation.

Compliance with Ethics Guidelines

Conflict of Interest

All authors (Bimal Patel, Surekha Pendyal, Priya Kishnani, Marie McDonald, and Lauren Bailey) declare there are neither competing interests nor financial disclosures.

Informed Consent

All procedures followed were in accordance with the ethical standards of the responsible committee on human experimentation (institutional and national) and with the Helsinki Declaration of 1975, as revised in 2000. Informed consent was obtained from the patient included in this study.

Animal Studies

This chapter does not contain any studies with animal subjects performed by the any of the authors.

Authorship Contributorship Statements

All authors have been involved in (a) conception and design, or analysis and interpretation of data, and (b) drafting the chapter or revising it critically for important intellectual content.

Table 1 Documented cases of subependymal nodules in patients with biochemical and genetic testing confirming glutaric acidemia type 1

	Proband	Herskovitz et al. (2013)	Korman et al. (2007)	Pierson et al. (2015)
Sex/background	Female, Caucasian	Male, Iraqi Jewish	Male, Palestinian Arab	Female, Hispanic Mexican
Age of diagnosis	2 months old	56 years old	30 years old	55 years old
Comorbidities	Idiopathic intracranial hypertension	None reported	None reported	Crohn's disease
Neurologic symptoms	Migrainous and IIH headaches, mild learning disability, recent onset slurred speech with left facial weakness/numbness	30-year history of pain in feet, gradual weakness in legs, speech disturbance, and incontinence	Borderline IQ, normal neurological exam; otherwise "asymptomatic"; discovered after seeking prenatal genetic counseling as he was paternal uncle of another patient in the case series	Bilateral lower extremity spasticity, numbness, and paresthesias
MRI findings	Callosal and periventricular white matter changes, age discordant parenchymal atrophy, and multifocal subependymal nodules (a type of heterotopia or disorganized brain tissue) in the lateral ventricles	Communicating hydrocephalous, bilateral frontotemporal atrophy, bilateral temporal arachnoid cysts, prominent periventricular and deep leukodystrophy, and subependymal cauliflower-like mass lesions	Patchy signal changes in the corpus callosum with wart-like mass lesions extending from the ependymal lining into the lateral ventricles in the upper part in the ventricular system and showing some contrast enhancement, resembling subependymal nodules found in tuberous sclerosis	Extensive bilateral white matter changes in the periventricular deep and subcortical white matter tracts; multiple subependymal nodules projecting into lateral ventricles; temporal lobe hypoplasia; normal striatum and corpus callosum
GCDH gene mutations	Homozygous for the c.1204 C>T, p.R402W pathogenic variant	Previously reported homozygous Gly101Arg mutation	Compound heterozygosity of a novel variant (c. 578_579 insTCA; pThr193_R194insHis) and known pathogenic mutation (c.877G>A; p.Ala293Thr)	Compound heterozygosity of a novel variant (c.1219 C>G; pLeu407Val) and known pathogenic mutation (c.848delT;pL283RfsX8)

All coauthors have seen the final version of the chapter, confirm that the work has not been published/submitted elsewhere, and agree with submission.

Bimal Patel:	conception and design, analysis, interpretation of data, writing/drafting of the manuscript, final approval of chapter.
Surekha Pendyal:	conception and design, analysis, interpretation of data, final approval of chapter.
Priya Kishnani:	primary physician caring for patient since early childhood, conception and design, analysis, interpretation of data, final approval of chapter.
Marie McDonald:	conception and design, analysis, interpretation of data, final approval of chapter.
Lauren Bailey:	genetic counselor caring for patient, conception and design, analysis, interpretation of data, final approval of chapter.

References

Biery BJ, Stein DE, Morton DH et al (1996) Gene structure and mutations of glutaryl-coenzyme A dehydrogenase: impaired association of enzyme subunits that is due to an A421V substitution causes glutaric acidemia type I in the Amish. Am J Hum Genet 59:1006–1011

Boy N et al (2017) Proposed recommendations for diagnosing and managing individuals with glutaric aciduria type I: second revision. J Inherit Metab Dis 40:75–101

Busquets C, Coll MJ, Ribes A (2000) Evidence of a single origin for the most frequent mutation (R402W) causing glutaryl-CoA dehydrogenase deficiency: identification of 3 novel polymorphisms and haplotype definition. Hum Mutat 15:207

Gupta N, Singh PK, Kumar M et al (2015) Glutaric acidemia type 1-clinico-molecular profile and novel mutations in GCDH gene in Indian patients. JIMD Rep 21:45–55

Herskovitz M et al (2013) Subependymal mass lesions and peripheral polyneuropathy in adult-onset glutaric aciduria type I. Neurology 81:849–850

Klar N, Cohen B, Lin DD (2016) Neurocutaneous syndromes. Handb Clin Neurol 135:570

Kölker S, Valayannopoulos V, Burlina AB et al (2015) The phenotypic spectrum of organic acidurias and urea cycle disorders. Part 2: The evolving clinical phenotype. J Inherit Metab Dis 38:1059–1074

Korman SH et al (2007) Glutaric aciduria type 1: clinical, biochemical, and molecular findings in patients from Israel. Eur J Paediatr
Neurol 11:81–89

Kuczmarski RJ, Ogden CL, Grummer-Strawn LM et al (2000) CDC
growth charts: United States. Adv Data 314:1–27

Pierson TM et al (2015) Adult-onset glutaric aciduria type I presenting
with white matter abnormalities and subependymal nodules.
Neurogenetics 16:325–328

Twomey EL, Naughten ER, Donoghue VB et al (2003) Neuroimaging
findings in glutaric aciduria type 1. Pediatr Radiol 33:823–830.
https://doi.org/10.1007/s00247-003-0956-z

JIMD Reports
DOI 10.1007/8904_2017_68

RESEARCH REPORT

Mitochondrial Trifunctional Protein Deficiency: Severe Cardiomyopathy and Cardiac Transplantation

C. Bursle · R. Weintraub · C. Ward · R. Justo ·
J. Cardinal · D. Coman

Received: 02 August 2017 / Revised: 17 October 2017 / Accepted: 19 October 2017 / Published online: 10 November 2017
© Society for the Study of Inborn Errors of Metabolism (SSIEM) 2017

Abstract We describe mitochondrial trifunctional protein deficiency (MTPD) in two male siblings who presented with severe cardiomyopathy in infancy. The first sibling presented in severe cardiac failure at 6 months of age and succumbed soon after. The second sibling came to attention after newborn screening identified a possible fatty acid oxidation defect. Dietary therapy and carnitine supplementation commenced in the neonatal period. Despite this the second child required cardiac transplantation at 3 years of age after a sudden and rapid decline in cardiac function. The outcome has been excellent, with no apparent extra-cardiac manifestations of a fatty acid oxidation disorder at the age of 7. Pathogenic *HADHA* mutations were subsequently identified via genome wide exome sequencing. This is the first reported case of MTPD to undergo cardiac transplantation. We suggest that cardiac transplantation could be considered in the treatment of cardiomyopathy in MTPD.

Communicated by: Saskia Brigitte Wortmann, M.D., Ph.D.

C. Bursle · D. Coman (✉)
Department of Metabolic Medicine, The Lady Cilento Children's
Hospital, Brisbane, QLD, Australia
e-mail: david.coman@health.qld.gov.au

C. Bursle · C. Ward · R. Justo · D. Coman
School of Medicine, University of Queensland, Brisbane, QLD,
Australia

R. Weintraub
Department of Cardiology, The Royal Children's Hospital,
Melbourne, VIC, Australia

R. Weintraub
School of Medicine, University of Melbourne, Melbourne, VIC,
Australia

C. Ward · R. Justo
Department of Cardiology, The Lady Cilento Children's Hospital,
Brisbane, QLD, Australia

J. Cardinal
Cardinal Bioresearch, Brisbane, QLD, Australia

D. Coman
Department of Paediatrics, The Wesley Hospital, Brisbane, QLD,
Australia

D. Coman
School of Medicine, Griffith University, Gold Coast, QLD, Australia

Introduction

The mitochondrial trifunctional protein (MTP, OMIM 609015) is an enzyme complex which catalyses the last 3 steps in the long chain fatty acid β-oxidation cycle (Houten and Wanders 2010). This protein complex comprises 4 α-subunits with enoyl CoA hydratase (LCEH) and 3-hydroxyacyl CoA dehydrogenase (LCHAD) activity and 4 β-subunits with 3 ketoacylCoA thiolase (LKAT) activity (Uchida et al. 1992). The α and β subunits are encoded by the *HADHA* (OMIM 600890) and *HADHB* (MIM 143450) genes, respectively (Kamijo et al. 1994), which both map to 2p22.3 (Yang et al. 1996).

MTP deficiency demonstrates a heterogeneous clinical spectrum including a severe neonatal form with cardiomyopathy, Reye-like features and early death; a hepatic phenotype with recurrent hypoketotic hypoglycaemia; and a milder later onset neuromyopathic type with episodic rhabdomyolysis (Boutron et al. 2011; den Boer et al. 2003). Mortality remains high, reported at 39% (LCHAD deficiency) to 76% (MTP deficiency) in the largest case series (Boutron et al. 2011; den Boer et al. 2002, 2003).

Cardiac involvement is common in long chain fatty acid oxidation defects (LC-FAOD) and is often a cause for mortality (Vockley et al. 2015; Baruteau et al. 2014). Cardiac presentations include arrhythmias, hypertrophic cardiomyopathy, dilated cardiomyopathy, left ventricular non-compaction cardiomyopathy, and even severe in utero hypertrophic cardiomyopathy (den Boer et al. 2003; Baruteau et al. 2014; Spiekerkoetter et al. 2008; Emura and Usuda 2003; Ojala et al. 2015). These clinical phenotypes bear resemblance to the cardiac manifestations of the mitochondrial respiratory chain defects (Yaplito-Lee et al. 2007) and represent a significant cause of morbidity.

Improvements in the care of children with cardiomyopathy, congenital heart disease and acquired heart disease have led to an increased number of children surviving with advanced heart failure (Alexander et al. 2014; Kindel and Everitt 2016). Key improvements include the development of left ventricular assist devices (LAD) and a clearer understanding of immunology in the prevention of transplant rejection (Zangwill 2017). Donor availability and thus suitable candidate selection remain challenges. Herein we describe the first case of MTPD to undergo cardiac transplantation.

Case Reports

These siblings are the product of a non-consanguineous union with two older healthy children. The ultimate diagnosis of MTP deficiency came via genome wide exome sequencing after sibling 2 had received a cardiac transplant.

Sibling 1 This previously well male infant presented at 6 months of age with an intercurrent viral respiratory illness, in cardiac failure secondary to severe dilated cardiomyopathy. He required intensive support including extracorporeal membrane oxygenation (ECMO). There were no other manifestations to suggest a multi-system disease or an infective process. Plasma acylcarnitine profile demonstrated persistently elevated long and medium chain fatty acylcarnitine species, i.e. tetradecenoylcarnitine C14 1.9 μmol/l (reference range < 0.7 μmol/l), tetradecanoylcarnitine C14:1 1.1 μmol/l (RR < 0.3), hexadecanoylcarnitine C16 1.1 μmol/l (RR < 0.6), decanoylcarnitine C10 0.8 μmol/l (RR < 0.4), octanoylcarnitine C8 0.3 μmol/l (RR < 0.2) and hexanoylcarnitine C6 0.3 μmol/l (RR < 0.2). The urine organic acids consistently demonstrated significantly raised levels of 3-hydroxydicarboxylic acids (C10 > C12, C8 and C6) with moderate dicarboxylic acids. Extended newborn screening (ENBS) was normal. ENBS was collected at 52 h of age while the child was clinically well and breast feeding in the maternity ward. Very long chain acyl-CoA dehydrogenase enzyme assay was normal, as were acylcarnitine studies performed on cultured fibroblasts were normal (performed in New South

Wales Biochemical Genetic Service, Lehman et al. 1990). This screening assay studies the acylcarnitine profile produced by intact cells in culture medium with added palmitate and carnitine, with the butylated acylcarnitine species detected by electrospray ionization tandem mass spectrometry. The latter result appeared inconsistent with the plasma and urine results. A cardiac biopsy demonstrated interstitial oedema and fibrosis, and mitochondrial respiratory chain analysis on a muscle biopsy demonstrated mildly reduced complex IV activity 2.16 (3.3–9.1/min/mg, performed in MCRI Mitochondrial laboratory). A long chain fatty acid oxidation defect was suspected, the patient was managed with carnitine supplementation (50–75 mg/kg/day), avoidance of prolonged fasting, and trialled triheptanoin at 1 g/kg/day which was not well tolerated due to palatability and diarrhoea. The child succumbed to cardiac failure at 9 months of age prior to a final diagnosis being forthcoming.

Sibling 2 The younger male sibling came to attention in the neonatal period after an abnormal ENBS result, with elevated long chain acylcarnitine species, i.e. elevated C14 1.29 (RR < 0.63 μM), C14:1 1.36 (RR < 0.6 μmol/l), 3-hyrdoxypalmitoylcarnitine (C16-OH), 3.2 (RR < 0.2 μmol/l). On this basis, as well as the family history, he was managed for a presumed fatty acid oxidation disorder with avoidance of fasting, carnitine supplementation (50–75 mg/kg/day) and medium chain triglyceride-based formula (Monogen 50 g twice daily). Urine organic acids and repeat plasma acylcarnitine profiles were normal. Mitochondrial respiratory chain studies performed on the explanted cardiac tissues were normal (performed in MCRI Mitochondrial laboratory). Sequencing of the *ACAD9* gene (Mater Pathology Brisbane), the *ACADVL* gene (Department of Biochemistry and Molecular Biology, Arhus University Hospital, Denmark), the common *HADHA* mutation c.1528G>C and a next generation sequencing cardiomyopathy panel of 69 genes (performed in Victorian Clinical Genetics Pathology Service, Victoria), all returned normal results.

At 3 years of age he developed severe dilated cardiomyopathy detected on routine monitoring, the left ventricle had dilated significantly to 51 mm, shortening fraction 21% and biplane ejection fraction 41%. Over the ensuing weeks he rapidly progressed toward congestive cardiac failure. Medical management including the use of Lisinopril and carvedilol. D-β-hydroxybutyrate (300 mg/kg/day) was attempted and while this generated a measurable ketoacidosis on urine testing, there was no appreciable improvement in cardiac function. A cardiac transplant was considered the only long-term option for survival. This was facilitated by the implantation of a left ventricular assist device followed by conversion to a Berlin heart. He required multiple explorations for bleeding and removal of thrombus from the cannula. He had a brief generalized tonic clonic seizure triggered by hypoxia in the context of pericardial tamponade. Neuroimaging at this time was normal. Orthotopic heart transplantation occurred 3 months after initiation of augmented circulatory supports, when suitable donor was available. Our recipient had become sensitized and was mismatched for Class I and II antigens by Luminex Single Antigen testing, as well as being CMV mismatched on serology (donor positive – recipient negative). The post-transplant course was complicated by lymphopenia secondary to mycophenalate motefil, mild rejection on endocardial biopsies, gastric bleeding due to a gastric ulcer, adrenal suppression secondary to steroid immune suppression and medical procedure anxiety. The patient is doing well at the age of 7. He is intellectually normal and has no signs of a multisystem disease process. Rather than repeating specific FAOD enzyme assays on cultured fibroblasts, we proceeded to whole exome sequencing. He is not on any specific metabolic management currently.

Whole Exome Sequencing

A trio-based clinical exome, and subsequent sanger sequencing, was performed in the Macrogen laboratories (http://www.macrogen.com/eng/). After enrichment of all the coding and flanking intronic regions of the genes mentioned above, sequencing analysis was performed using an Illumina HiSeq platform. 97.7% of targeted regions achieved ×100 coverage and 99.7% achieved ×10 coverage. The only clinically relevant sequence variations with an allele frequency <0.1% were HADHA NM_000182 c.1712T>C; p.Leu571Pro. (maternal), and HADHA NM_000182 c.446G>T; p. Gly149Val (paternal). The variants have not been previously reported on dbSNP. Minor/alternative allele frequencies are not reported in the 1000 genome or the NHLBI GO Exome Sequencing Project data sets at either of these loci. *HADHA* NM_000182 c.1712T>C; p.Leu571Pro, overlaps with evolutionary constrained element (detected using SiPhy-ω and SiPhy-π statistics). The conservation across 28 species is described with PhyloP (score: 2.33). GERP identifies constrained elements in multiple alignments by quantifying substitution deficits (score: 6.07). The BLOSUM62 substitution matrix reports a score of −3 for this alteration, with a PhyloP score of 2.33 and aGERP score of 6.07. HADHA NM_000182 c.446G>T; p. Gly149Val, variant overlaps with evolutionary constrained element (detected using SiPhy-ω and SiPhy-π statistics). The BLOSUM62 substitution matrix reports a score of −3 for this alteration. The conservation across 28 species is described with a PhyloP score of 1.47 and GERP score of 4.94. Both are predicted to be missense mutations.

Discussion

The pathophysiology of severe, early onset cardiac phenotypes in MTPD is unclear, but provide an indication that the heart is exquisitely sensitive to impaired LC-FAOD, either due to direct toxicity from metabolic accumulation, or from substrate deficiency. The heart undergoes a switch in energy substrate preference from glucose in the foetal period to fatty acids following birth (Spiekerkoetter et al. 2008; Lehman and Kelly 2002). However; the in utero onset of cardiac manifestations in some MTPD cases suggests a pathogenic role in mitochondrial respiratory chain (MRC) function or permeability (Ojala et al. 2015; Tonin et al. 2013; Nsiah-Sefaa and McKenzie 2016).

The beta-oxidation pathway and the MRC share substrates and are linked biochemically. Reduced NAD and FADH2 produced during fatty acid oxidation pass their electrons to the MRC complexes. Primary disorders of one of these pathways have been shown to have deleterious effects on the other (Nsiah-Sefaa and McKenzie 2016), from the build-up of toxic intermediates (Sakai et al. 2015) or physical links between beta-oxidation and MRC protein complexes (Taylor et al. 2012; Nouws et al. 2014). MTP is bound to MRC complex 1 (Sumegi and Srere 1984), suggesting that beta-oxidation-MRC super-complexes are metabolically active structures (Nsiah-Sefaa and McKenzie 2016). Patients with LCHAD deficiency frequently exhibit secondary MRC complex 1 deficiencies (Tyni et al. 1996; Das et al. 2000; Wang et al. 2010), either via physical interaction (Wang et al. 2010), or altered stability via cardiolipin (Taylor et al. 2012). The extreme severity of the neonatal mitochondrial cardiomyopathies, rapidly fatal in a majority of cases, clearly illustrates the major role of myocardial MRC function in the adaptation to extrauterine life (Schiff et al. 2011). The heart relies heavily on oxidative metabolism and is particularly vulnerable to MRC dysfunction (Yaplito-Lee et al. 2007). The consequences of MRC dysfunction include ATP deficiency, aberrant calcium handling, excessive reactive oxygen species production, apoptosis dysregulation and nitric oxide deficiency (Yaplito-Lee et al. 2007).

Subject one demonstrated normal ENBS results despite being collected in appropriate physiological conditions. German experience with newborn screening for MTP defects in 1.2 million infants reports 11 true positives, 10 false positive but no known false negative results (Sander et al. 2005). However, two false negatives were reported in Austrian LCHAD deficient twins who were born prematurely (29 weeks gestation) and supplemented with L-carnitine (Karall et al. 2015). Intermittently normal acylcarnitine profiles have been reported in cases of later onset neuromyopathic MTPD deficiency (Yagi et al. 2011).

Though a diagnosis of fatty acid oxidation was strongly suspected based on the clinical and biochemical parameters, the diagnosis of MTPD was not formalized when decision-making was required regarding the suitability of sibling 2 as a cardiac transplantation candidate. He demonstrated single organ disease and was of normal intellectual and developmental capabilities. While concerns of cardiac dysfunction secondary to "toxic metabolites" are a possibility in the LC-FAOD, we proposed that the LC-FAOD cardiac clinical phenotypes maybe secondary to substrate deficiency as outlined above, and recurrence in a transplanted heart would not be expected. Possible evidence of substrate depletion being causative is demonstrated by sibling 2's different clinical trajectory after management from birth with metabolic supportive therapy and anaplerotic treatments consequent to his abnormal ENBS. The role of anaplerotic therapy in the LC-FAOD, specifically triheptanoin, is under ongoing investigation (Vockley et al. 2015).

Our patient remains metabolically stable 4 years post cardiac transplantation with no apparent MTPD-related extra-cardiac manifestations such as retinitis pigmentosa, peripheral neuropathy, hepatic disease or neurological disease. However, long-term follow-up will be required as these complications may occur later in life.

Conclusion

In summary, we present the first case of cardiac transplantation in a defect of the mitochondrial trifunctional protein. The outcome in this case has been excellent, and while long-term complications related to the underlying fatty acid oxidation defect may occur despite dietary therapy, our experience suggests that transplantation could be considered to treat severe cardiomyopathy in this disorder.

Synopsis

Cardiac transplantation could be considered in the treatment of cardiomyopathy in mitochondrial trifunction protein deficiency.

Contributors' Statements

Dr. Carolyn Bursle is a metabolic fellow involved in patient care and development of the manuscript.

Drs. David Weintraub, Cameron Ward and Robert Justo are paediatric cardiologists involved in patient care and manuscript development.

Dr. John Cardinal is a medical scientist involved in manuscript development.

Professor David Coman is a metabolic physician involved in patient care and has driven the manuscript design and development.

All authors approved the final manuscript as submitted and agree to be accountable for all aspects of the work.

Corresponding Author

David Coman.

Conflict of Interest

The other authors have no conflicts of interest to disclose.

Funding Source

This project was supported by the Kevin Milo Benevolent Fund.

Ethics Approval

N/A.

Patient Consent

The patients' parents consent to publication of this case report.

References

Alexander PM, Swager A, Lee KJ et al (2014) Paediatric heart transplantation in Australia comes of age: 21 years of experience in a national centre. Intern Med J 44(12a):1223–1231
Baruteau J, Sachs P, Broué P (2014) Clinical and biological features at diagnosis in mitochondrial fatty acid beta-oxidation defects: a French pediatric study from 187 patients. J Inherit Metab Dis 37(1):795–803
Boutron A, Acquaviva C, Vianey-Saban C et al (2011) Comprehensive cDNA study and quantitative analysis of mutant HADHA and HADHB transcripts in a French cohort of 52 patients with mitochondrial trifunctional protein deficiency. Mol Genet Metab 103(4):341–348
Das AM, Fingerhut R, Wanders RJ et al (2000) Secondary respiratory chain defect in a boy with long-chain 3-hydroxyacyl-CoA dehydrogenase deficiency: possible diagnostic pitfalls. Eur J Pediatr 159(4):243–246
den Boer MEJ, Wanders JA, Morris AAM et al (2002) Long-chain 3-hydroxyacyl-CoA dehydrogenase deficiency: clinical presentation and follow-up of 50 patients. J Pediatr 109:99–104

den Boer ME, Dionisi-Vici C, Chakrapani A et al (2003) Mitochondrial trifunctional protein deficiency: a severe fatty acid oxidation disorder with cardiac and neurologic involvement. J Pediatr 142 (6):684–689

Emura I, Usuda H (2003) Morphological investigation of two sibling autopsy cases of mitochondrial trifunctional protein deficiency. Pathol Int 53(11):775–779

Houten S, Wanders R (2010) A general introduction to the biochemistry of mitochondrial fatty acid β oxidation. J Inherit Metab Dis 33:469–477

Kamijo T, Aoyama A, Komiyama A et al (1994) Structural analysis of cDNAs for subunits of human mitochondrial fatty acid β-ocidation trifunctional protein. Biochem Biophys Res Commun 199:818–825

Karall D, Brunner-Krainz M, Kogelnig K et al (2015) Clinical outcome, biochemical and therapeutic follow-up in 14 Austrian patients with long-chain 3-hydroxy acyl CoA dehydrogenase deficiency (LCHADD). Orphanet J Rare Dis 10:21

Kindel SJ, Everitt MD (2016) A contemporary review of paediatric heart transplantation and mechanical circulatory support. Cardiol Young 26(5):851–859

Lehman JJ, Kelly DP (2002) Transcriptional activation of energy metabolic switches in the developing and hypertrophied heart. Clin Exp Pharmacol Physiol 29(4):339–345

Lehman TC, Hale DE, Bhala A, Thorpe C (1990) An acyl-coenzyme A dehydrogenase assay utilizing the ferricenium ion. Anal Biochem 186(2):280–284

Nouws J, Te Brinke H, Nijtmans LG et al (2014) ACAD9, a complex I assembly factor with a moonlighting function in fatty acid oxidation deficiencies. Hum Mol Genet 23(5):1311–1319

Nsiah-Sefaa A, McKenzie M (2016) Combined defects in oxidative phosphorylation and fatty acid β-oxidation in mitochondrial disease. Biosci Rep 36(2):e00313

Ojala T, Nupponen I, Saloranta C et al (2015) Fetal left ventricular noncompaction cardiomyopathy and fatal outcome due to complete deficiency of mitochondrial trifunctional protein. Eur J Pediatr 174(12):1689–1692

Sakai C, Yamaguchi S, Sasaki M et al (2015) ECHS1 mutations cause combined respiratory chain deficiency resulting in Leigh syndrome. Hum Mutat 36(2):232–239

Sander J, Sander S, Steuerwald U et al (2005) Neonatal screening for defects of the mitochondrial trifunctional protein. Mol Genet Metab 85:108–114

Schiff M, Ogier de Baulny H, Lombès A (2011) Neonatal cardiomyopathies and metabolic crises due to oxidative phosphorylation defects. Semin Fetal Neonatal Med 16(4):216–221

Spiekerkoetter U, Mueller M, Cloppenburg E et al (2008) Intrauterine cardiomyopathy and cardiac mitochondrial proliferation in mitochondrial trifunctional protein (TFP) deficiency. Mol Genet Metab 94(4):428–430

Sumegi B, Srere PA (1984) Complex I binds several mitochondrial NAD-coupled dehydrogenases. J Biol Chem 259(24):15040–15045

Taylor WA, Mejia EM, Mitchell RW et al (2012) Human trifunctional protein alpha links cardiolipin remodeling to beta-oxidation. PLoS One 7(11):e48628

Tonin AM, Amaral AU, Busanello EN et al (2013) Long-chain 3-hydroxy fatty acids accumulating in long-chain 3-hydroxyacyl-CoA dehydrogenase and mitochondrial trifunctional protein deficiencies uncouple oxidative phosphorylation in heart mitochondria. J Bioenerg Biomembr 45(1–2):47–57

Tyni T, Majander A, Kalimo H et al (1996) Pathology of skeletal muscle and impaired respiratory chain function in long-chain 3-hydroxyacyl-CoA dehydrogenase deficiency with the G1528C mutation. Neuromuscl Disord 6(5):327–337

Uchida Y, Izai K, Orii T et al (1992) Novel fatty acid β-oxidation enzymes in rat liver mitochondria. J Biol Chem 267:1034–1041

Vockley J, Marsden D, McCracken E et al (2015) Long-term major clinical outcomes in patients with long chain fatty acid oxidation disorders before and after transition to triheptanoin treatment – a retrospective chart review. Mol Genet Metab 116(1–2):53–60

Wang Y, Mohsen AW, Mihalik SJ et al (2010) Evidence for physical association of mitochondrial fatty acid oxidation and oxidative phosphorylation complexes. J Biol Chem 285(39):29834–29841

Yagi M, Lee T, Awano H et al (2011) A patient with mitochondrial trifunctional protein deficiency due to the mutations in the HADHB gene showed recurrent myalgia since early childhood and was diagnosed in adolescences. Mol Genet Metab 104:556–559

Yang BZ, Heng HH, Ding JH et al (1996) The genes for the alpha and beta subunits of the mitochondrial trifunctional protein are both located in the same region of human chromosome 2p23. Genomics 37(1):141–143

Yaplito-Lee J, Weintraub R, Jamsen K et al (2007) Cardiac manifestations in oxidative phosphorylation disorders of childhood. J Pediatr 150(4):407–411

Zangwill S (2017) Five decades of pediatric heart transplantation: challenges overcome, challenges remaining. Curr Opin Cardiol 32(1):69–77

JIMD Reports
DOI 10.1007/8904_2017_69

RESEARCH REPORT

Three Cases of Hereditary Tyrosinaemia Type 1: Neuropsychiatric Outcomes and Brain Imaging Following Treatment with NTBC

Helen Walker · Mervi Pitkanen · Yusof Rahman ·
Sally F. Barrington

Received: 22 April 2017 / Revised: 18 October 2017 / Accepted: 23 October 2017 / Published online: 16 November 2017
© Society for the Study of Inborn Errors of Metabolism (SSIEM) 2017

Abstract *Aim*: To examine neuropsychiatric outcomes in adults with hereditary tyrosinaemia type I (HT-1), treated with 2-(2-nitro-4-trifluoromethylbenzoyl)-1,3-cyclohexane-dione (NTBC) and correlate these with functional imaging as well as with tyrosine and phenylalanine-tyrosine (Phe: Tyr) ratios.

Design: We retrospectively reviewed the medical records of three adult HT-1 patients with a particular focus on their FDG PET/CT brain scans, neuropsychiatric assessment (including neurocognitive assessment and mood and anxiety ratings) as well as mean tyrosine and phenylalanine levels and Phe:Tyr ratios for 3-month period. The patients had been referred to a specialist joint inherited metabolic disorder and neuropsychiatry clinic. They were all on NTBC; two since 6 weeks of age, and one since 9 years of age.

Results: All patients performed below the expectation on the formal neurocognitive testing and had raised plasma tyrosine levels and reduced plasma Phe:Tyr ratios. FDG PET/CT-brain scans were normal in two patients and the third patient (treated with NTBC from 6 weeks) had reduced metabolism in temporal and medial frontal areas bilaterally which correlated with the neurocognitive performance.

Conclusions: All three HT-1 patients treated with NTBC had high tyrosine levels, reduced Phe:Tyr ratios and under-performed in neurocognitive testing regardless of the point when the NTBC was first started. One had imaging abnormalities which also correlated with neurocognitive performance. The patient who struggled the most in neuro-cognitive testing had the highest average plasma tyrosine levels and the lowest Phe:Tyr ratio. Overall, these cases appear to support the previous hypothesis that either the high tyrosine levels or abnormal phenylalanine hydroxylase (PAH) function may well be the causative factor for poor neurocognitive performance. Further systematic, multi-centre studies with a longer follow-up are required to further clarify the relationship between HT-1, NTBC treatment, tyrosine and phenylalanine levels and neurocognitive outcomes.

Communicated by: John Christodoulou, MB BS PhD FRACP FRCPA

H. Walker
West London Mental Health Trust, London, UK
e-mail: Helen.walker43@nhs.net

M. Pitkanen (✉)
Department of Neuropsychiatry and Memory Disorders,
King's College London, London, UK
e-mail: mervi.pitkanen@kcl.ac.uk

Y. Rahman
Centre for Inherited Metabolic Disorders, Guy's and St Thomas'
Hospital NHS Foundation Trust, London, UK

S.F. Barrington
KCL and Guy's and St Thomas' PET Centre, King's College London,
King's Health Partners, St. Thomas' Hospital, London, UK

Introduction

HT-1 is a rare genetic disease caused by mutations in the gene for the enzyme fumarylacetoacetase, and typically present in early infancy with acute liver failure. It can also manifest as chronic liver dysfunction, cirrhosis, neurological crisis and occasional renal tubular dysfunction with hypophosphataemic rickets. Without treatment, patients with HT-1 have a high lifetime risk of developing hepato-cellular carcinoma (HCC), resulting from the cytotoxicity of tyrosine metabolites accumulating proximal to the metabolic defect. NTBC was first used in the early 1990s for the treatment of HT-1 and has transformed the natural history of tyrosinaemia. NTBC acts on tyrosine metabolism upstream of the defect and is used in combination with a tyrosine- and phenylalanine-restricted diet.

However, recent studies have hypothesised that along with improving the overall survival, the treatment with NTBC may increase the likelihood of neurocognitive impairment (Bendadi et al. 2014; De Laet et al. 2011; Masurel-Paulet et al. 2008; Thimm et al. 2011, 2012; Ginkel et al. 2016). Some suggest that this neurocognitive decline may be mediated by increased plasma and CSF tyrosine but clear association between IQ and tyrosine levels have not yet been demonstrated.

Previous studies which include brain imaging are inconclusive. A small case series demonstrated normal MRI brain scans in HT-1 patients treated with NTBC (Thimm et al. 2011, 2012), yet another study confirmed brain abnormalities on the MRI (high signal changes in the globus pallidus and high signal changes in the posterior limbs of the internal capsules) in two young HT-1 children treated with NTBC (Sener 2005a, b). An animal study (Sgaravatti et al. 2008) supported a potential aetiological role of hypertyrosinaemia in cognitive decline caused by NTBC treatment, reporting that the elevated tyrosine levels resulted in DNA damage in the cerebral cortex of young rats attributable to a decrease in enzymatic and non-enzymatic antioxidant defences.

Interestingly, the majority of HT-1 studies have focused on neurocognition in children and generally have limited their investigations to IQ testing. Although it has been proposed that hypertyrosinaemia is a potential aetiological factor in neurocognitive decline, studies of HT-1 patients treated with NTBC are small and literature on adult outcomes is still sparse. Hence, there is a pressing clinical need to further understand the long-term neurocognitive implications of treatment with NTBC. This study was designed to further investigate the neurocognitive outcomes in HT-1 adult patients, as opposed to children, by employing more extensive neuropsychiatric investigations and comparing these with plasma and Phe:Tyr ratios as well as with FDG PET/CT brain imaging.

Methods

Three patients with HT-1, treated with NTBC, and seen in a specialist neuropsychiatry clinic for patients with inherited metabolic disorders between August 2011 and October 2011 were examined; neuropsychiatric assessment, blood testing and FDG PET/CT brain scans were conducted for each patient. Blood tests were based on averaged results for a period of 3 months prior to the brain scans. No ethics committee permission was required as this was considered a retrospective anonymised audit of clinical practise.

Functional Neuroimaging

PET scans were performed in the PET Imaging Centre at St Thomas' Hospital, using a GE Discovery ST PET/CT scanner (GE Medical Systems, Milwaukee, WI, USA) with a 15.7 cm axial field of view. Participants were instructed to refrain from eating or drinking anything except plain water for 3 h prior to the scan. On arrival each participant was injected with 250 MBq [18F]-FDG. After a 30-min uptake period during which they rested in a dimly lit quiet room, the participants were positioned on the PET scanner, with their head secured by a head rest. A planar CT scout was acquired to localise the participant's brain in the PET field of view; then a single low dose CT was acquired for attenuation correction of the PET scan. The PET scan was acquired as a single frame for 15 min. Images were reconstructed using OSEM iterative reconstruction. The images were displayed in three orthogonal planes scaled to the maximum activity concentration and visually interpreted by two experienced PET readers and later re-reviewed for the purposes of this report to confirm the accuracy of the findings.

Neuropsychiatric Assessment

Participants were assessed on a subset of the following standardised neuropsychological measures: estimated optimal adult intellectual functioning (National Adult Reading Test, NART, Wechsler Test of Adult Reading, WTAR or Test of Premorbid Functioning, TOPF); current intellectual functioning (Wechsler Abbreviated Scale of Intelligence, WASI, or Wechsler Adult Intelligence Scales, WAIS); memory (Doors and People, Camden Memory Test or Wechsler Memory Scales, WMS); naming (Graded Naming Test), visual perception and visuospatial functioning (Visual Object and Space Perception battery, VOSP); arithmetic (Graded Difficulty Arithmetic Test); executive functioning (Behavioural Assessment of Dysexecutive Syndrome, BADS, Hayling and Brixton Tests, Modified Wisconsin Card Sort, Trail-Making, Verbal Fluency); manual dexterity (Purdue Pegboard). Assessments took place in a quiet room in an outpatient clinic as part of routine clinical care.

Subjective cognitive difficulties were assessed by using standardised questionnaires (Prospective and Retrospective Memory Questionnaire, PRMQ, Dysexecutive Questionnaire, DEX) as were mood and anxiety symptoms (Beck Depression Inventory II, BDI-II or Hospital Anxiety and Depression Scale, HADS). Participants were asked to rate their health and quality of life on a 10-point Likert scale (0 worst, 10 best).

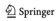

Biochemical Investigation

Blood tests were carried out to ascertain mean tyrosine and phenylalanine levels and Phe:Tyr ratios over a period of 3 months.

Case Descriptions

Patient 1 was a 16-year-old white British male, who complained of memory problems which he thought impacted on his school performance. Two days after birth he had developed septicaemia and meningitis and on his 6th week was diagnosed with HT-1, and NTBC with a low protein diet was commenced. His motor developmental milestones had been normal but his verbal milestones were reported as delayed. At assessment he was on NTBC 30 mg am and 40 mg nocte with a restricted natural protein diet of 23 g per day and 3 of TyrCooler 20® supplements per day. He had vitamin B12 deficiency (59 ng/L) which was a result of poor compliance with his fortified TyrCooler 20®.

Patient 2 was a 19-year-old British Indian male who complained of memory problems. He was diagnosed with HT-1 at infancy and began NTBC treatment at 6 weeks of age. His speech and motor developmental milestones were broadly within normal limits. At assessment he was on NTBC 20 mg twice a day with a restricted natural protein diet of 15–18 g per day, and 3 of TyrCooler 20® supplements per day. He had history of Vitamin D and B12 deficiency (undetectable and 151 ng/L respectively).

Patient 3 was a 24-year-old white non-British male who complained of memory problems impacting his learning and work. He had suffered from mild liver dysfunction during the first year of his life. At the age of four he had presented with rickets hypophosphatasia of his lower limbs and was subsequently diagnosed with HT-1. He was commenced on NTBC at the age of 9; however, due to the limited availability of the drug he was only on a low dose until the age of 13. He continued to suffer from symptoms of rickets due to phosphate loss caused by renal tubolopathy. At assessment he was on NTBC 40 mg twice a day with a low natural protein diet. He was diagnosed with clinical depression and was prescribed fluoxetine.

Results

Neuropsychological Testing

Neuropsychological testing results are summarised in Table 1. A detailed summary of neuropsychological testing can be found in Appendix.

Patient 1: performance was impaired on tests of perceptual motor function, mixed on tests of executive functioning and average on tests of memory.

Patient 2: performance was largely in the average range in intellectual functioning and in line with his estimated premorbid functioning but borderline impaired (1–2 SDs below the mean) on processing speed, semantic memory and cognitive flexibility. He was not anxious or depressed

Table 1 Neuropsychological testing (percentile ranks)

| | | | Memory | | Frontal | | | | |
| | | | | | | | | Delis Kaplan executive function system | |
Patient	Premorbid IQ	Full-Scale IQ	Visual	Verbal	Trail A	Trail B	Perdue pegboard	Visual scanning	Number and letter sequencing and number-letter switching
1	104	83	21	45	10	40	<0.1	Not completed	Not completed
2	99	86	25	75	25–50	10–25	Not completed	Not completed	Not completed
3	92	Verbal comprehension index: 76 Perceptual organisation index: 86	<1	9	Not completed	Not completed	<0.1	37	<0.1

and he rated his health and quality of life as good (9/10) and rated his subjective memory as good.

Patient 3: performance was impaired in intellectual functioning, working memory, verbal recall, visual recognition, executive function and perceptual motor function but in the borderline range for verbal comprehension, processing speed and visual recall. He rated himself as depressed and anxious with poor health (3/10) and poor quality of life (2/10) but he did not think he had memory problems (Table 2; Figs. 1 and 2).

Table 2 Neuroimaging and haematological results

Patient	FDG PET/CT scan result	Tyrosine level (μmol/L)	Phenylalanine level (μmol/L)	Phe: Tyr ratio
1	Normal	595.9	48.9	0.08
2	Bilateral temporal and medial frontal hypometabolism	611.6	58.5	0.10
3	Normal	760.1	55.1	0.07

Discussion

Previous studies have largely focussed on changes in IQ and have been inconclusive with heterogenous results. Our case series employed a detailed neuropsychiatric assessment, reviewed recent plasma tyrosine levels and Phe:Tyr ratios as well as FDG PET/CT brain imaging in order to achieve a more comprehensive understanding of the effects HT-1 and NTBC treatment may have on adult patients.

Neurocognitive testing did not reveal a clear pattern of deficits but confirmed that all three HT-1 patients underperformed in cognitive testing, regardless of the point when the NTBC treatment was first started. The abnormal functional neuroimaging result for one patient demonstrated consistency with his neurocognitive performance but this patient also had severe vitamin D and B12 deficiencies which may well have contributed to his neurocognitive underperformance.

All the patients had raised tyrosine levels, which may support the hypothesis that hypertyrosinaemia is implicated in the declined neurocognitive functions. The oldest patient (patient 3) performed least well, had the highest tyrosine level and the lowest Phe:Tyr ratio. However, when interpreting his cognitive performance on testing one should

Neuroimaging

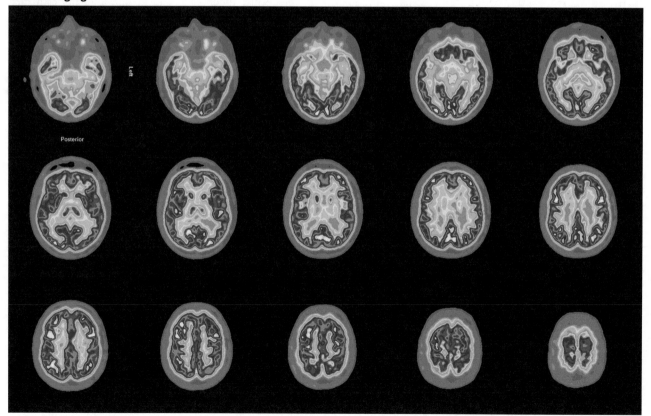

Fig. 1 Patient 1: Normal scan

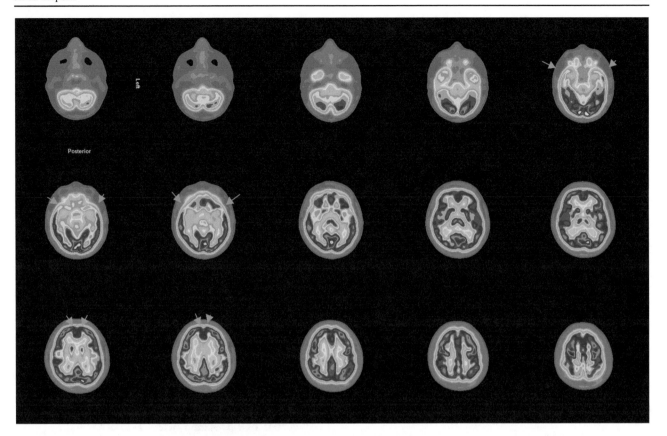

Fig. 2 Patient 2: Abnormal scan showing bilateral temporal and medial frontal hypometabolism (arrows)

note that his first language was not English and he was also clinically depressed.

Previous small case series have demonstrated inconsistent MRI brain imaging findings in HT-1 patients. This study, using functional brain imaging, FDG PET/CT scan, demonstrated two normal scans and one with abnormalities.

Although our case series has limitations given the small sample size, it is the first one which compares neurocognitive performance with blood tests (tyrosine and Phe:Tyr ratio) and functional brain imaging and appears to confirm that there is a relationship between HT-1 and neurocognitive compromise. However, due to the study limitations we are unable to draw any conclusions which of these investigations are more sensitive to detect functional impairment. Further systematic, longitudinal, multi-centre studies are necessary in order to understand the relationship between HT-1, NTBC treatment and neurocognitive outcome and the relationship between tyrosine and phenylalanine levels and cognitive decline.

Appendix

Patient 1

IQ

Predicted Full Scale IQ (National Adult Reading Test): 104. Full Scale IQ (WAIS): 83.

Memory

Wechsler Memory Scale IV

WMS IV domain	Percentile rank
Auditory memory	21
Visual memory	45
Visual working memory	58
Immediate memory	19
Delayed memory	39

Frontal-Executive Function

Verbal Fluency: 37th percentile.

Hayling and Brixton tests

Domain	Percentile rank
Hayling Part A (time)	25
Hayling Part B (time)	50
Hayling Part B (errors)	50
Brixton test (errors)	75

Trail Making Test

Part A: 10th percentile.
    Part B: 40th percentile.

Manual Dexterity

Perdue pegboard

Domain	Percentile rank
Dominant hand	5
Non-dominant hand	<0.1
Both hands	5
Assemblies, both hands	<0.1

Patient 2

IQ

Predicted Full Scale IQ (National Adult Reading Test): 99.
    Full Scale IQ (WAIS): 86.

Memory

Doors and People

Domain	Percentile rank
People (verbal recall)	25
Doors (visual recognition)	10–25
Shapes (visual recall)	75
Names (verbal recognition)	10–25

Frontal-Executive Function

Verbal Fluency: 63rd percentile.

Hayling and Brixton tests

Domain	Percentile rank
Hayling Part A (time)	50
Hayling Part B (time)	50
Hayling Part B (errors)	50
Brixton test (errors)	50

Trail Making Test

Part A: 25–50th Percentile.
    Part B: 10–25th Percentile.

Patient 3

IQ

Predicted Full Scale IQ (National Adult Reading Test): 92.
    Full Scale IQ (WAIS): Could not be measured due to lack of consistency within the Verbal Comprehension Index and clinically significant differences between the Verbal and Performance Indexes.
    Verbal Comprehension Index: 5th percentile.
    Perceptual Organisation Index: 18th percentile.
    Working Memory Index: <1st percentile.
    Processing Speed Index: 5th Percentile.

Memory

Doors and People test

Domain	Percentile rank
People (verbal recall)	<1st percentile
Doors (visual recognition)	<1st percentile
Shapes (visual recall)	9th percentile
Names (verbal recognition)	16th percentile

Frontal-Executive Function

Delis-Kaplan executive function system – trail making test

Domain	Percentile rank
Visual scanning	37
Number sequencing	<0.1
Letter sequencing	<0.1
Number-letter switching	<0.1
Motor speed	25

Delis-Kaplan executive function system – verbal fluency test

Domain	Percentile rank
Letter fluency	9
Category fluency	5
Category switching total	9
Category switching accuracy	9

Modified Wisconsin Card Sorting task

Domain	Percentile rank
Total errors	60
% perseverative errors	20

Worrington Graded Calculation test: <5th Percentile.

Manual Dexterity

Perdue pegboard

Domain	Percentile rank
Dominant hand	38
Non-dominant hand	8
Both hands	4
Assemblies	<0.1

Details of the Contributions of Individual Authors

Dr. Helen Walker (corresponding author): Drafting of the chapter, conception and design, and analysis and interpretation of data.

Dr. Pitkanen: Critical review, conception and design, analysis and interpretation of data.

Dr. Rahman: Critical review, conception and design, analysis and interpretation of data.

Dr. Barrington: Critical review, conception and design, analysis and interpretation of data.

Funding

This research received no specific grant from any funding agency in the public, commercial or not-for-profit sectors.

Conflict of Interest

The authors declare that they have no conflict of interest.

Consent

Informed consent was obtained for all participants included in the study.

Guarantor

Dr. Mervi Pitkanen.

References

Bendadi F, de Koning TJ, Visser G, Prinsen HCMT, de Sain MGM, Verhoeven-Duif N, Sinnema G, van Spronsen FJ, van Hasselt PM (2014) Impaired cognitive functioning in patients with tyrosinaemia type I receiving nitisinone. J Pediatr 164:398–401

De Laet C, Terrones Munoz V, Jaeken J, Francois B, Carton D, Sokals EM, Dan B, Goyens PJ (2011) Neuropsychological outcome of NTBC-treated patients with tyrosinaemia type 1. Dev Med Child Neurol 53:962–964

Masurel-Paulet A, Poggi-Bach J, Rolland MO, Bernard O, Guffon N, Dobbelaere D, Sarles J, de Baulny HO, Touati G (2008) NTBC treatment in tyrosinaemia type I: long-term outcome in French patients. J Inherit Metab Dis 31:81–87

Sener RN (2005a) Tyrosinaemia: computed tomography, magnetic resonance imaging, diffusion magnetic resonance imaging, and proton spectroscopy findings in the brain. J Comput Assist Tomogr 29:323–325

Sener RN (2005b) Brain magnetic resonance imaging in tyrosinaemia. Acta Radiol 46:618–620

Sgaravatti ÂM, Vargas BA, Zandoná BR, Deckmann KB, Rockenbach FJ, Moraes TB et al (2008) Tyrosine promotes oxidative stress in cerebral cortex of young rats. Int J Dev Neurosci 26(6):551–559

Thimm E, Herebian D, Assmann B, Klee D, Mayatepek E, Spiekerkoetter U (2011) Increase of CSF tyrosine and impaired serotonin turnover in tyrosinaemia type I. Mol Genet Metab 102:122–125

Thimm E, Richter-Werkle R, Kamp G, Molke B, Herebian D, Klee D, Mayatepek E, Spiekerkoetter U (2012) Neurocognitive outcome in patients with hypertyrosinaemia type I after long-term treatment with NTBC. J Inherit Metab Dis 35:263–268

van Ginkel WG et al (2016) Neurocognitive outcome in tyrosinemia type 1 patients compared to healthy controls. Orphanet J Rare Dis 11(1):87

Printed in the United States
By Bookmasters